ILLUSTRATIONS

OF

MADNESS

Tavistock Classics
in the History of Psychiatry

GENERAL EDITORS:

W.F. Bynum and Roy Porter

Current interest in the history of psychiatry is growing rapidly both among the psychiatric profession and social historians. This new series is designed to bring back into print many classic documents from earlier centuries. Each reprint has been chosen for the series because of its social and intellectual significance, and includes a substantial introduction written by an eminent scholar in the history of psychiatry.

Life's Preservative Against Self-Killing (c.1637)
by John Sym (*ed.* Michael MacDonald)

An Essay . . . on Drunkenness (1804)
by Thomas Trotter (*ed.* Roy Porter)

Observations on Maniacal Disorders (1792)
by William Pargeter (*ed.* Stanley W. Jackson)

ILLUSTRATIONS

OF

MADNESS

BY

JOHN⌊HASLAM

Edited with an Introduction by

Roy Porter

R

ROUTLEDGE
London and New York

First published 1988
by Routledge
11 New Fetter Lane, London EC4P 4EE
29 West 35th Street, New York, NY 10001

© 1988 Introduction by Roy Porter

Printed in Great Britain at the University Press, Cambridge

British Library Cataloguing in Publication Data

Haslam, John
    Illustrations of madness.
    1. Medicine. Psychiatry – Case studies
    I. Title   II. Porter, Roy, *1946* –
    III. Series
    616.89′09

Library of Congress Cataloging in Publication Data

Haslam, John, 1764–1844.
    Illustrations of madness/John Haslam; edited with an
introduction by Roy Porter.
        p.   cm. — (Tavistock classics in the history of psychiatry)
    Reprint. Originally published: London: Printed by G. Hayden.
1810.
    ISBN 0–415–00637–6
    1. Mathews, James Tilly—Mental health.   2. Mentally ill—Great
Britain—Biography.   3. Mental illness—Case studies.   I. Porter,
Roy, 1946– .   II. Title.   III. Series.
    [DNLM: 1. Mathews, James Tilly.   WM H349i 1810a]
RC464.M379H37 1988
616.89—dc19
DNLM/DLC   88–18631
for Library of Congress   CIP

ISBN 0–415–00637–6

CONTENTS

v

PREFACE

The Tavistock Classics in the History of Psychiatry series meets a
considerable need amongst academics, practitioners, and all those
who are more broadly interested in the development of psychiatry.
Psychiatry as a discipline has always paid considerable heed to its
own founders, its history, and emergent traditions. It is one field in
which the relevance of the past to the present does not diminish.
There is a high professional awareness of the history of the subject,
and many aspects of this are now benefiting from fruitful dialogue
with the now rapidly expanding investigations of historians and
historical sociologists.

Yet two factors greatly hamper our grasp of psychiatry's past. On
the one hand, a considerable number of the formative texts in the
rise of psychiatry are exceedingly difficult to obtain, even from
libraries. As a small discipline in earlier centuries, many of the major
works were published only in small runs, and many, even of the
classics, have never been reprinted at all. This present series aims to
overcome this problem, by making available a selection of such key
works. Mostly they are books originally published in the English
language; in other cases where the original language was, say, French
or German, we are reprinting contemporary English translations; in
a few cases, we hope to present entirely new translations of classic
Continental work.

On the other hand, in many instances little is commonly known
of the life and ideas of the authors of these texts, and their works
have never been subjected to thorough analyses. Our intention in
this series is to follow the model of the now defunct Dawson series
of psychiatric reprints, edited and introduced by Richard Hunter

and Ida Macalpine, now, alas, both dead, and to provide substantial scholarly introductions to each volume, based upon original research. Thus the book and its author will illuminate each other, and one will avoid the dilemma of a text isolated in an intellectual vacuum, or simply the accumulation of miscellaneous biographical data. It is our hope that this series will break new ground in the history of psychiatry, and secure a new readership for a number of illustrative works in psychiatry's rich and fascinating past.

ACKNOWLEDGEMENTS

The materials held in the Bethlehem Archives have been made available by kind permission of the Bethlehem Royal Hospital and the Maudsley Hospital Health Authority. For their help both in source material research and in interpreting this case I am deeply grateful to Patricia Allderidge, Jonathan Andrews, Ben Barkow and Dorothy Porter.

ACKNOWLEDGMENTS

INTRODUCTION

Roy Porter

The cardinal premise of psychiatry, its *raison d'être* and *sine qua non*, is the claim that reason can diagnose, understand and treat madness. There can be no psychiatry – or at least none which does not risk becoming a travesty – unless it can be reliably established that it is one of the powers, indeed privileges, of sound mind to be able to identify the insane. Jeopardize the reality of this polar distinction between reason and unreason, mental health and mental disorder, and the very state of psychiatry totters.

Of course, the experience of common people, doctors and magistrates through history has ordinarily been unproblematic in this respect. The presence of the raving, axe-swinging maniac, foaming at the mouth, the drooling simpleton, the anguished suicidal depressive, tormented by delusions of fiends and hellfire, or of the autistic sinister schizophrenic hardly sows scepticism about what Roth and Kroll have recently called 'the reality of mental illness', even if the aetiology and nosology of such mental maladies remain profoundly mysterious even today.[1] From the Greeks onwards, it was confidently believed that lunacy unambiguously revealed itself by its physical appearance, behaviour and speech-patterns,[2] and over the last couple of centuries, specialist psychiatric doctors have developed sophisticated diagnostic methods of detecting the modes of madness.

But the situation has never in reality been so simple. For one thing, certain traditions in western culture, while not denying the reality of insanity, have sought to evaluate certain expressions of it, not as a disease or a disability, but rather as a blessing when manifest, for example, in the ecstatic saint or the mad genius. Hence being mad was not necessarily being bad or sad, but a state possibly divine or at least desirable, rendering the moral boundary between sanity and insanity somewhat ambiguous.[3] For another, it has often been contended that there is, or can be, reason in madness and madness in reason. Just as *in vino veritas*, so the words, thoughts and deeds of the lunatic or fool might afford their own superior insights. Thus it was a common jest in early modern England that the inmates (or 'collegians') of Bedlam – London's Bethlem Hospital (i.e., what was more properly known as the Bethlehem Hospital) – were the truly rational folks, protected against the masses of madmen peopling the nation at large: a point suggested in the Bedlam scene which concludes Hogarth's 'Rake's Progress'.[4] Acknowledging such traditional perceptions, certain recent historians, sociologists and 'anti-psychiatrists', most notably Thomas Szasz, have argued that we must cease to regard the sane/insane divide as either self-evident or as medico-scientifically proven, and instead treat these antithetical categories as social constructs. In this view, 'insanity' would be seen as a label imposed by those in authority upon various deviant groups for the purposes of stigmatization, professional aggrandizement and social control.[5]

Of course, doubts about the diagnostic *differentiae* of madness become specially crucial in deciding the fate of the individual case. Before the eighteenth century it was probably the exception rather than the rule in Britain and elsewhere in Europe for lunatics to be placed under formal legally-enforceable institutional detention: as late as 1700, Bethlem, which held little more than a hundred patients, remained the only public lunatic asylum in the whole of the British Isles.[6] This situation changed, however. During the eighteenth century both charitable and private asylums were instituted, and in the nineteenth century these were augmented by a comprehensive system of county asylums. Between 5,000 and 10,000 people were confined as lunatics by 1800, and about 100,000 by 1900.[7]

As ever larger numbers of people were thus confined, and thereby lost the exercise of their liberty and civil rights, the question of proper certification procedures necessarily stirred public concern.[8] In Britain these long remained casual; under an Act of 1714, pauper lunatics could be detained on the authority of a magistrate, while families continued to be able to lodge supposedly insane relatives in private asylums without the need for any formal authorisation at all, by either a JP or a medical practitioner. The inmate's only possible redress lay in a suit of habeas corpus, which for obvious reasons was not a ready recourse, though it did prove successful on a few occasions. As confinement grew in the Georgian age, so a patients' protest literature began to appear alongside it. Ex-inmates alleging they had been wrongfully held protested in print to Parliament and posterity – witness Alexander Cruden's *The London Citizen Exceedingly Injured* (London, 1739).[8a]

Stronger safeguards were first introduced by the Madhouses Act of 1774, which applied to private asylums. This stipulated that confinement would henceforth be legal only when legitimated by a certificate of insanity provided by a medical practitioner. Of course this provision might be said to cut both ways. It could protect the sane patient against arbitrary confinement by unscrupulous relatives, eager to seize property or to nullify an unfavourable will. On the other hand, the existence of such a certificate – possibly obtained after only a rather cursory examination by a doctor with no special psychiatric expertise – could sanction protracted, and even lifelong, detention.[9]

Individual cases continued to attract publicity in which the insanity of the patient, and hence the propriety of confinement, was challenged. Almost immediately after the passing of the 1774 Act, the Stamford tradesman Samuel Bruckshaw rushed into print with his *The Case, Petition and Address of Samuel Bruckshaw* (London, 1774),[9a] and his *One More Proof of the Iniquitous Abuse of Private Madhouses*,[9b] published in the same year, alleging that he had been locked up – though perfectly sane – as a consequence of a villainous conspiracy hatched by his commercial rivals. Comparable accusations of malicious confinement form the burden of William Belcher's *Address to Humanity, Containing a Letter to Dr Munro, a Receipt to Make a Lunatic, and Seize his Estates, and a Sketch of a True Smiling Hyena* (London, 1796).[10] The nefarious imprisonment of the sane in 'English Bastilles' formed a prominent theme in Gothic horror novels, and continued to produce *causes célèbres* in real life down into Victorian times.[11]

In some ways more perturbing, however, were cases of contested lunacy in which bad faith played no part. What when a patient protested his sanity but the mad-doctors testified to his insanity? Or, more perplexing still, when the supposedly mad patient could count upon the witness of friends, relatives, and even of medical practitioners themselves, as to his own sanity? Such an eventuality obviously challenged that very ontological divide between reason and madness upon which psychiatry hinged.

This dilemma becomes increasingly severe from the turn of the nineteenth century. This was for two reasons. First, there was a new tendency to confine lunatics not merely – as formerly – if they were a positive danger to themselves or to others, but rather simply because they were insane, in the belief, fostered by a new climate of therapeutic optimism, that they would recover with proper treatment. For that reason there was a growing likelihood that the cases in dispute would centre upon people showing less florid symptoms of madness than typical formerly.[12] Second, developments within psychiatry were leading to enlarged notions of latent or partial insanity or, later, J. C. Prichard's idea of 'moral insanity'. These varieties would, it was said, often be invisible to the untrained or lay eye, though quite conspicuous to the expert psychiatrist. James Parkinson argued along these lines in his *Madhouses* (1811), in connexion with the case of a contested patient, Mary Daintree. Her family claimed she was sane and requested her release. Leaning on his authority and experience as a practitioner, Parkinson responded by maintaining that appearances were deceptive; remission might be only temporary, relapses were common, that it was the prime duty of the certifying physician to protect the public at large, even at the risk of erring on the side of caution.[13]

Thus by the early nineteenth century the possibility had arisen that the signs and symptoms of insanity might dissolve into a veritable will-o'-the-wisp. Indeed, the parallel with the emperor's new clothes suggested itself: were those doctors who saw insanity rampant everywhere merely seeing things? The implications of these uncertainties constitute, of course, the core of the radical challenge to the psychiatric enterprise over the last two centuries – a questioning induced not least by supposedly mad patients themselves. What guarantee is there that the 'mad' are truly suffering from mental disease? For might not their 'madness' be a rational response by the patient to a threatening, even crazy, world – one in which psychiatry itself may be experienced as one of the threats? Or might it even be a 'projection' of the distorted psychiatric imagination?[14] Doubts such as these provide the background to the protracted war waged between John Haslam, apothecary to Bethlem Hospital, and James Tilly Matthews, one of his patients, in the first decades of the nineteenth century.

Matthews was confined in Bethlem as a lunatic, indeed eventually as an 'incurable lunatic'. He protested his sanity, and his family, friends and parish authorities petitioned for his release. The medical staff of Bethlem insisted that he always had been, and remained, quite insane, and felt so strongly on this issue that Haslam was moved to pen a whole volume, the *Illustrations of Madness* (1810), to clinch the point; he thereby produced the first book-length case study of a single patient in British psychiatric history. Yet there is something disturbing, both in tone and substance, about Haslam's own performance; and through making an enemy of the possibly quite harmless if extremely odd Matthews, Haslam ended up by heaping coals upon his own head. Matthews's fate became a *cause célèbre*; it was used against Bethlem in general and Haslam in particular when the institution came under the scathing scrutiny of the House of Commons committee investigating madhouses in 1815;[15] and when the governors of Bethlem felt obliged to review Haslam's conduct, documents written by Matthews, alleging maltreatment, weighed heavily with them, leading to Haslam's dismissal in 1816. Thus the lunatic Matthews proved rational enough, or at least cunning enough, to outwit the man who wrote a book to prove him mad. These issues will be investigated in greater detail below. But first it will be useful to provide brief background sketches of the lives of Matthews and Haslam, before considering the problems raised by the text of Haslam's *Illustrations of Madness*.

James Tilly Matthews

James Tilly Matthews was a tea-broker of 84 Leadenhall Street in London. He was Welsh in origin; his mother, a Tilly, came of French Huguenot stock. Nothing is known of his early life.[16] Anxious in the early 1790s about the deterioration of Anglo-French relations, he developed extensive contacts with his countryman, the radical intellectual, David Williams, who was friendly with Girondin leaders such as Brissot and Le Brun. Williams had begun to act as a go-between on behalf of the French, in the hope of preventing a

British declaration of war. Matthews, who in these early years represented himself as a 'republican', supported these endeavours. From 1792, in a series of missions from Paris to London, he attempted to communicate peace overtures to Pitt and other ministers: Pitt refused to see him, though apparently he had an audience with Lord Grenville. When the Jacobins came to power, Matthews fell under suspicion – partly because of his Girondin sympathies, partly because it was believed he was a double agent. He was arrested in 1793, and held until 1796, during which time the authorities apparently concluded he was a 'dangerous lunatic', and eventually released him (in his autobiography Williams reports that even from 1792 he had 'suspicions that Matthews was affected in the head').[17] At some point during his French stay Matthews seems to have become interested in Mesmerism, which was still fashionable despite the enforced departure of Mesmer from the capital in 1784, following the unfavourable report of the investigating Commission set up by Louis XVI.

On his release, Matthews, returned to England in March 1796. By then his mind had obviously become profoundly disordered by the intense danger, disturbances and machinations of the years passed in gaol, presumably under constant threat of execution. Our next record of his activities is contained in a letter he wrote to Lord Liverpool on 12 September 1796. I have preserved its spelling and punctuation, so as not to endow it with a spurious coherence:[18]

> Your Lordship will well remember, in the first days of May in the year ninety three, I had the honor of an interview with your Lordship at Addiscombe Place, in which I made known to your Lordship the certainty I had of being able to effect a total change of Principles and Measures, then pursuing, or adopted in France. I communicated also to your Lordship and demanded your Lordships Assistance in the efforts I was then making to open a door for Accommodation between the two Nations. I remember well the pleasure your Lordship seemed to enjoy at the prospect of returning reason in a country from which, the Commercial Interests of Great Britain, and the honor of his Majesty's Crown, both so dear to your Lordship could derive true lustre and advantage: and I confess to your Lordship it acted upon me as a Stimulus to push with additional Vigour the

project I had formed of becoming Instrumental in effecting that Change – The Circumstances which took place in France a few weeks afterwards, namely the General Proscription of Talents and the triumph of anarchy by the insurrection of the 31 May, seemed as if purposely wrought in contradiction to all the assurances which I had been making of the desire of those who became the Victims, to restore honor and peace to their distracted Country, and to Cultivate friendship with Great Britain. It necessitated my instant return to Paris where I became equally the object of intrigue and every other measure which could be devised seemed practised, in order to entrap and destroy me: It was even pretended in faithless secrecy that persons of Consequence in this Country, and [illegible] if true Your Lordship must shudder, were giving information to those in power, that I had hostile views, and even agency from the British Gouvernment – think then my Lord what was my Situation! However it happens that I am not frightened soon by a whole Jacobin Army! On the contrary, convinced that by perseverance my efforts must be successful, I even made another journey to London for the purpose of urging the possibility, and of preventing Great Britain from becoming the dupe to the Treason of some of its Allies! I returned to France for the powers which had been promised me to act fully and officially, after having given assurance of the readiness of France to accede to honorable Conditions, and to save the unfortunate Family then in the Temple. But in coming and returning my Lord the hand of perfidy every where was behind me. I have since been informed often, and even till my leaving France, that there were treacherous men in England, connected with the Monsters of France, whose Intrigues had even extended to Counteract every effort of mine. Poor infatuated Jealousy! so it has appeared. At the moment I was offering the safety of the unhappy Marie Antoinette (or within Ten days afterwards), she was dragged from the Temple to the Conciergerie, and the mislead multitude were prepared to ask for her death. I reached Paris as soon as possible after frustrating some attempts to prevent me; and I had hopes of saving the unfortunate Princess and family: I was even promised from day to day full powers to act; when at the very moment I was expecting to receive them I was put in

Arrestation and a law which had been expressly passed two days before, was intended to take away my life. I was charged with being the particular Confidant of your Lordship; – the disaster of Toulon at that moment hardly made public, as well as all the misfortunes which had befallen France were laid to my charge. Letters were fabricated pretendedly found on the ramparts of Lisle, at St Omas etc discovering plots centred in me, the distribution of Agents and money throughout France etc etc, when it was on behalf of France particularly that I was exerting myself to restore peace. When all this had been so far arranged as to have a plausible pretence of putting me to death, an offer was held out to me of Ten Millions Livres Tournois if I should join in a plan to stir up Insurrections in Great Britain; an atrocious set were associated for this purpose. I refused, and of course became subject to all the Vengeance of those inveterate Enemies of the British name. I pursued my plan; admonished and preached up the renowned honor of the court of St James's: as I proceeded thus pamphlets were published, written speeches were pronounced, and all that malignant invective could offer was committed by such miserables against the persons of the King and his August family, as also against the Constitution of Great Britain: – It pleased Heaven to assist, Events and the Vigour of the British Parliament had destruction among them; – one party was annihilated, another struck with fear: these returned to their usual protestations of Sincerity, and were the first to pretend detestation of the atrocities which they had Committed. On my part I had tenders of Riches and honor, Palaces even to join them; by my Lord I detest assassins the veriest Enemies of every thing British who in their adversity wo.d flatter, but in the day of propriety wo.d destroy it. I was then thrown into prison, (for till now a space of fifteen months, I had been in custody of Gendarmes) – Secret information was given me, that very large sums of money had ben delapidated, as well as valuables, as it had been pretended by those in power that such sums had passed through my hands, and been appropriated to the promotion of Insurrection in England; But my Lord, these as well as inestimable treasures which had been plundered from the unfortunate Victims sacrificed by those monsters, had been expended, in part no doubt among miscreants of Confusion in England, as well in their own immoral pleasures; but principally in order to induce Prussia to betray its engagements and in the Insurrections in Poland, all which were but too fully verified by the Conquest of Holland and the peace with Prussia. Such sums and valuables it seemed were inquired after. As it was a custom too common with those beings, wherever any favorable Circumstance to their arms took place, to boast among their Friends of their dextrous management in the way of Corruption, and thus take all the merit to themselves; fearing their infamy sho.d be carried so far as to charge the British Gouvernment with having sacrificed its duty, and thus permitted the Conquest of Holland, and prolonged the war by conniving at the atrocities which were thus but too likely to have been received, I resolved rather to perish wanting food than suffer the British name to be wounded at least with my Consent; – I therefore refused all the offers w.h were continually held out to me equally despising their Guillotine and their Palaces. Full Fourteen Months I continued to be dragged from Prison to Prison, and being continually reduced in wretchedness, till at last, after continual remonstrances and approaches, as well to the Councils of Legislature, as to all the Ministers; but especially the Directory, I was conducted on foot from Paris to Calais by the Gendarmes, in that state of misery, that I made many of the stages barefooted; had not covering sufficient to preserve my nakedness from the intense cold; conducted from dungeon to dungeon and in many places refused Bread to eat, experience even personal violence from my instructed Conductors I sh.d say from one in particular, for by some I was even fed. But my Lord I experience all this as an Englishman; still refusing all offers, and came to England in such Circumstances, and for the reasons given. It was the 21st August 1793 when I last entered France, and the 9th March 1796 when I landed in England. While this had happened to me in France other measures to destroy me had been put in practice in England: a Communication had been issued ag.t me, and I was outlawed; but this was not all, for on finding here my distressed family, I learnt that sometime towards the end of Ninety Three, four or five Persons had committed a forgery on the Bank of England, and much pains had been taken to spread abroad that it was me; although I can with truth aver, that I never heard the name but of one, and him I never saw but four or five times. Certainly it was expected I could never escape the snares laid before me, and that my Death must render detection impossible – I have taken the necessary measures in my power, being without pecuniary means, to show the atrocity of the injuries with which I have been loaded, but as there seems to be much evasion, I shall think myself to publish to all the world every transaction which has come to my knowledge, and of w.h I have the most positive information. It is on these Grounds that I have omitted addressing your Lordship before. Nevertheless I have communicated to the Minister the General Grounds w.h may be made the pacification of Europe, of these of course your Lordship is well acquainted. If you Lordship think it useful, I will do myself the honor of calling at your Lordship's office at Whitehall, or at Addiscombe Place; and explain to your Lordship further how such a desirable Event may be perfected. I have the honor to be my Lord

    Your Lordships mo. do.t. Hble Sert
    James Tilly Matthews

Unfortunately there is no record as to how Lord Liverpool responded to this farrago about plots and persecution, from which it is difficult to sift a core of truth (which is presumably that Matthews had indeed suffered great privations in France under acute threats to his life) from the tissue of fantasy. Presumably the meeting which Matthews requested did not in fact take place. Thereafter there is no information about his activities until he wrote a follow-up letter to Lord Liverpool on 6 December 1796, which runs:[19]

My Lord
As your Lordship is but too well acquainted with my History, it would be loosing time to enter into it. What I have to say to your Lordship here will be short, but unfortunately true, of this your Lordship in Conscience, and soon I hope the Public at large, will admit. I pronounce your Lordship to be in every sense of the word a most diabolical Traitor. – After a long life of Political and real iniquity, during which your Lordship by flattering and deceiving, and more than anyone contributing to

deceive your King, who believing your hypochictical Professions, has to the detriment of many of the Countries Friends loaded you with honours, and Emoluments, you have made yourself a principal in Schemes of Treason founded upon the most extensive Intrigue, and which have not only long since laid your Country at the feet of its most bitter Enemies, those who have assassinated France; but even comprised Projects, which after having put every Branch of the Royal Family without exception either directly or indirectly in motion to Counteract or undermine each other, have absolutely aimed at the death of your benefactor, to reap further Advantages from those who by such wickedness might in such General Assassinating scramble mount the throne. After having by every possible means counteracted me in the effort to save Louis Seize; by means of those infamous Men of France, who forming a Corresponding Committee of the Convention; were in connexion with the Secret Cabinet in the Court of St James's, of which you have been the Prime Mover, you did actually affect the murder of that unfortunate Monarch – under their promise of placing upon the throne of France the Duke of York, you provoked and compassed the War, invited even the Enemy to invade your Country in the hope of being able in the Panic of fear and alarm to place your son at the Helm of Affairs: for this Purpose no efforts were wanting to render Nul every effort of mine as well before the War was declared to preserve, as after its declaration to restore Peace between England and France. You and your fellow labourers in iniquity caused the Insurrection in Paris on the Thirty First of May Ninety Three, which then, and at subsequent times in Consequence proscribed, or held in daily fear, every man who had been Consenting to support the Establishment of Order and good Gouvernment, as a base to Permanent Harmony between the two Countries. Such Intrigues also compassed the Murder of the unhappy Marie Antoinette, the Princess Elizabeth, & Louis dix Sept. You had already been an accomplice in receiving the Jewels of these [illegible] victims – now you deprived them of life to preserve Possession on the one part, and to put your own scholars in their places on the other. And as to myself who sought only the honour of rendering France and England as much Friends as they had usually been Rivals, Enemies; you in England and your Associates in France have caused both Nations to be Assassinated to deprive me of existence. They caused Toulon to be given up as arranged between you, to sacrifice me to popular fury; and you brought about for bribes its Evacuation, in order to support them in power. It was by such concealed Plans, and to prevent those Friends of England from showing themselves who from time to time have been ready to support my plans, that the [words cancelled] Austrian Army was obliged to Evacuate the Netherlands, and to effect which, with the Subsequent Evacuation of Holland, which was given up to be plundered, that the British Army was made to suffer continual defeats, till by such Treachery its remains became covered with [illegible] instead of the laurels which proper conduct must inevitably have procured it. It was the Secret Cabinet of Great Britain which counteracted the Negotiations set on foot with the Court of Vienna after the Evacuation of Belgia. – which permitted the retaking, and guaranteed possession to the French Gouvernment of the Colonies in the West Indies so to be retaken! – which caused the inaction of the British Army in Westphalia; – which after having by a Second and Counterplot to its first projects set on foot Schemes of Marriage between the Prince of Wales and the daughter of Louis Seize; and in Consequence been accessory to the Murder of the Brother of that innocent Princess, who after the Possession of the jewels had been received, was herself duped; – undertook to bring about the miscarriage of the expeditions to the coast of France! – which caused to be affected, the Price of all the necessary Articles of life in the markets of England; – and the fomenting of Insurrections in the different parts of England, Ireland and Corsica, to answer the Purposes, and for the support of the Counter Cabinet in France. – which caused to be betrayed into their hands the Commercial [illegible] of Great Britain – which connived at inaction and Rebellion in the British Colonies – which engaged to betray the British Fleets – to give up Gibraltar – to procure Successes to the French Arms etc etc Yes my Lord, although I was led from Paris under such Circumstances, I had information conveyed to me before I reached St Denis, that Spain was to declare War against England; to defeat the British Fleet and to take possession of Gibraltar etc – I am sorry my Continual Cries during nine months have not been able to prevent such Treason altogether. But my Lord, even if all this had been disinterested, it might have been Palliated under the appearance of at least misconduct only: but it has been for bribes that all this has been done – The Royal Family in its different Branches, Persons in attendance upon them, some Administrators, in office which have received Sums of Money, Diamonds and other jewels at different times and by Various Channels to the amount within my knowledge of upwards of three Millions but which I have had the most positive Assurance has amounted to upwards of four Millions Sterling – It is this my Lord which has commanded such Treason; which has effected such Events; and you are a Principal in such abominable iniquity – but even here it has not ended; for in later times, as I refused all connivance and connexion, German favours, Spanish honors, you would have given me the the Crown of France to have acquiesced in your Projects of bartering the wealth of the King of England to gratify the Extravagance of those Profligates who expected to succeed him – You my Lord have been privy to the Ambitious and Counteracting Projects of every Branch of the Royal Family, and with more than one such Branches you have encouraged the desire to destroy each other, and to accomplish the ruin, the Death even of all those whom you have found inimical to your crafty plans. Nor are you more free from Guilt with respect to the secret Machinations of the Emigrants, who for the protection which they experience, are but too many of them guilty of something more than ingratitude – but I have said enough here, and heretofore I hope to defeat the Machinations of those who to attain Gold or Jewels, to satisfy their love of Titles, or their Appetite for Emoluments, would establish in England the Inquisition of Spain, the Assassinating Committees of France, the Military Regime of Prussia, or in fact the Gouvernment of the Grand Turk, was there but a prospect of becoming Grand Vizier – I profess myself to be at open war with you my Lord, and with all those your partners or Apostles in craft and Treason. You may succeed in imposing upon the World that I am insane but I will persevere till I convince you and the World that I am perfectly otherwise. I hope my Lord that ere long the Country

will Judge impartially between us: meantime I have the honour
to subscribe myself My Lord,
      Your Lordship's mo. ob.t Sert.
      James Tilly Matthews

Once again, we do not know Liverpool's response to Matthews's
missive, which, with its convoluted accusations of treason, appears
more disturbed than the earlier letter, and which, through its
pugnacious closing sentences, seems to anticipate its reception.
Matthews almost seems to will Liverpool to engineer his eventual
fate ('you may succeed in imposing upon the world that I am
insane'), while maintaining a pathetic faith in the public as arbiter, in
hoping to convince the World 'that I am perfectly otherwise': the
challenge that 'the country will Judge impartially between us' did
not have the consequences Matthews expected.

Matthews soon proceeded to the gallery of the House of Commons
where he accused the ministry of 'traitorous venality', as Williams
put it. Hauled before the Privy Council, he was examined, as a
result of which his parish, Camberwell, was informed by the Lord
Chancellor that he should be not allowed at large. He was committed
to Bethlem on 28 January 1797. His family protested, but, after an
examination before Lord Kenyon, their protests were overruled.[20]

There Matthews remained. At the end of his first year he was
transferred to the incurable wing. Little is known of his condition,
except that in 1809 he and his relatives applied for his release on the
grounds that he was sane, and that the damp conditions in the
hospital were destroying his physical health.[21] It was at this point
that his relationship with John Haslam became critical.

John Haslam

Haslam was the apothecary to Bethlem, a job roughly equivalent to
being resident medical officer. Born in London in 1764, few details
survive of his early years.[22] He had a period as a medical apprentice,
moving on to St Bartholomew's Hospital where he attended George
Fordyce's lectures and became the pupil of Dr David Pitcairn. From
1785 he spent two years studying medicine at Edinburgh University
– he was a contemporary of Thomas Beddoes – and he proved

energetic in the student medical societies. The surviving disserta-
tions he delivered before the Royal Medical Society there already
reveal that brusque dismissiveness towards theory and abstract
speculation which marked his medical temper throughout his career. It
is probable that he went on to study for a time at Uppsala, before
settling into medical practice in London towards the close of the
1780s. He married, and a son was baptized in Shoreditch in 1790.

Nothing is then known of his career till he was appointed apothecary to Bethlem in 1795. He was to hold the post for twenty-one of
the most traumatic years in its history, being involved, *inter alia*, in
its move in 1815 from the palatial but collapsing Moorfields building to the new one in Lambeth (which houses the present Imperial
War Museum).

Haslam's working position at Bethlem was slightly ambiguous.
He formed one of a three-man medical team. There was a physician,
who was Dr Thomas Monro, the third member of that Monro
dynasty which was to dominate Bethlem under the Georges. The
physician received but £100 a year, about a third of the salary of the
apothecary; his post was assumed to be somewhat ceremonial.
Indeed, it appears that Thomas Monro visited the hospital perhaps
no more than once a month, and was certainly not involved in its
day-to-day running. A man more interested in water-colours than
in insanity, Monro was a supine figure, who made few attempts to
improve the regime inherited from his father, Dr John Monro.

Bethlem also had a surgeon, who for much of Haslam's period
was Bryan Crowther. Crowther, who himself had succeeded his
father in his post, was no medical nonentity, and he published some
pioneering post-mortem studies of the brains of lunatics.[23] In his
later years, however, he became an alcoholic, and eventually a
lunatic; as Haslam revealed to the House of Commons committee
on madhouses in 1815, for ten years Crowther, who continued in
post, was 'generally insane and mostly drunk. He was so insane as
to have a strait-waistcoat'.[24]

With the dubious support of an absentee physician and a mad
surgeon – one who (Haslam said) 'continued to pursue me with the
rankest hostility', believing that he had savagely reviewed one of his
books – Haslam became willy-nilly the sheet-anchor of the medical
establishment at Bethlem, although lacking formal standing and
authority. Initially he lived in, but, as the old Moorfields structure

crumbled, he moved to Islington, visiting the Hospital each morning. As apothecary, his post was not intended to be primarily psychiatric in nature – he was meant to attend to the general physical health of the patients. But the burdens of the overall therapy inevitably, if rather unfairly, devolved upon him.

The shortcomings, indeed evils, of Bethlem's medical regime were relentlessly exposed by the Commons committee of 1815; it was revealed, for example, that certain patients were kept naked, chained to the walls. Two particular individual scandals were exploited by reformers. One was the case of Matthews himself, to be examined below. The other was that of James Norris. Norris was an American sailor, allegedly a homicidal maniac, who had been permanently held for fourteen years in a complicated custom-built harness which almost wholly denied him movement. By the time reformers discovered him in 1814, Norris was a shrivelled, weak old man close to death. Under cross-questioning, Haslam described him as 'the most malignant and the most mischievous lunatic I ever saw in my life'; quizzed about the restraining apparatus, he shuffled between absolving himself from all responsibility for it, and complacently, though unconvincingly, defending it as comfortable, humane and therapeutic.[25]

Indeed, in much of his evidence Haslam displayed a counter-productive combination of cynicism, truculence and arrogance ('I have not been disposed to listen to those who had less experience than myself'). In displaying a seeming lack of concern for the plight of the inmates he misjudged the zeal of the reformers' onslaught against Bethlem's old regime.[26] His responses – autocratic, hostile, blustering and evasive – created a bad impression; to save their own faces the governors had little option but to require both Monro and Haslam to defend their conduct.

As mentioned above, Haslam's post at Bethlem was not a psychiatric one. He could hardly, however, be effective resident practitioner at Bethlem for nearly a generation without developing opinions about madness and its treatment. Such views were spelt out in a series of volumes, beginning in 1798 with *Observations on Insanity, with Practical Remarks on the Disease and an Account of the Morbid Appearances on Dissection*, a work republished at twice the original length in 1809 as *Observations on Madness and Melancholy, including Practical Remarks on those Diseases*. In 1810

Illustrations of Madness came out, and that was followed by *Considerations on the Moral Management of Insane Persons* in 1817, *Medical Jurisprudence* in the same year – it was the first work of forensic psychiatry in English – *Sound Mind* (1819), *A Letter to the Right Honourable, the Lord Chancellor, on the Nature and Interpretation of Unsoundness of Mind, and Imbecility of Intellect* (1823), and *On the Nature of Thought* (1835). Amidst this string of publications, Haslam twice defended his own professional conduct in print, in his *Observations of the Physician and Apothecary of Bethlem Hospital, upon the Evidence taken before the Committee of the Hon. House of Commons for Regulating Mad-Houses* (1816), and again in his *A Letter to the Governors of Bethlem Hospital, Containing an Account of their Management of that Institution for the last Twenty Years* (1818).

Historians of psychiatry have credited Haslam with giving the first precise clinical accounts of general paresis and of schizophrenia. This is not the place to evaluate these claims,[27] but they do point to an authentic feature of his writings – the fact that they abound in empirical observations upon individual cases, and in shrewd evaluations of these, while eschewing general theory. He radically distrusted claims made by psychiatrists to be able to comprehend at a fundamental level the essence of madness; such overweening ambition would be the height of folly, amounting almost to a professional delusion of grandeur. As he expressed it in connexion with the duties of a forensic witness:[28]

> If it should be presumed that any medical practitioner is able to penetrate into the recesses of a lunatic's mind, at the moment he committed an outrage; to view the internal play of obtruding thoughts, and contending motives – and to depose that he knew the Good and Evil, Right and Wrong he was about to commit, it must be confessed that such knowledge is beyond the limits of our attainment.

Haslam had a robust distrust of flights of medical speculation; he deflated the humbug of dressing up ignorance and nonsense in 'highfalutin' professional jargon. Indeed, he almost regarded theorizing about madness as a form of madness itself. Thus, in his first work, in his usual caustic style, he asked, apropos of attempts by his contemporaries to lay down foundations for psychiatry,[29] where is the elucidation of these general principles to be sought; and, in what manner are they to be applied according to the character, varieties, and intensity of madness? Is the work of Dr Arnold otherwise remarkable than as a burdensome compilation, or a multiplication of scholastic divisions, more calculated to retard than advance the progress of Science? Does Dr Harper, who announces in his preface, that he has quitted the beaten track, fulfil his promise in the course of his work? and is his section on mental indications any thing but a prolix commentary on the doctrines of the ancients? [and so forth]

Despite the nosologies of Thomas Arnold, proprietor of the Leicester asylum, Haslam believed that comprehensive taxonomies of madness were quite worthless. Insanity was better seen as a single basic disorder, visible in a variety of phases and manifestations. Sceptical even to the point of cynicism, it might prima facie seem as though Haslam were a John Bull figure, dismissive of the entire psychiatric enterprise. But that is not so. True, he had little faith in abstract schemes for explaining the nature, origin and phenomenology of insanity, and little confidence in the possibility of a general theory of mind. But he was convinced of the fundamental distinction between sound and unsound minds, and was a staunch advocate of practical psychiatry, believing in the capacity of the experienced practitioner, possessed of proper control and ascendency, to give beneficial treatment to the mentally sick. Though placing little faith in medicines, Haslam espoused what has been called 'moral management',[30] as he emphasised in his *Considerations on the Moral Management of Insane Persons* (1817).

But to note Haslam's attachment to moral management is not to suggest that he was some kind of humanitarian, advocating the virtues of kindness and gentleness; less still that he saw the mad either as pathetic victims or even as objects of pity. He was never inclined to regard lunatics other than as dreadful, often grotesque, and even laughable (there is a coarse humour even in the very title of the volume under consideration); they commonly possessed, he stressed, a low cunning, a deviousness of the will; they were untrustworthy, difficult, awkward and often dangerous. His fundamental axiom was that insanity was real; responsible practitioners owed it to society to expose madness in its true nature. The alienist who fudged that issue – who (for example) in the witness-box started apologising for, even rationalizing, the crimes of the mad – was himself betraying reason.

Matthews, Haslam and the *Illustrations of Madness*

These considerations must be borne in mind if we are to understand why the Matthews case agitated Haslam so profoundly, indeed, we might almost say, haunted him.

In 1809 Matthews's family, friends and parish petitioned for his release on the grounds that he had recovered his sanity. Rebuffed by the Bethlem authorities, they took out a suit of habeas corpus at the court of King's Bench. Seeking medical witnesses to his recovery, they engaged two London practitioners, George Birkbeck and Henry Clutterbuck, to examine him. These found him basically sane, although suffering from delusions on a few points; believing him safe they recommended his release.[31] Several other witnesses made depositions as to Matthews's sanity; one, Robert Dunbar, claimed that Haslam himself had informed him over a drink the previous year that Matthews 'never now touched upon those subjects but that he was perfectly quiet'.[32] Haslam, who together with Dr Thomas Monro was convinced, from having observed Matthews for over a decade, that he was quite mad, testified that Matthews always had been insane and so remained.[33] He claimed that Matthews's political delusions were such that, if released, he would be a danger to the Royal Family, the government and the public at large. Other witnesses endorsed Haslam's views. Richard Baldwyn, a governor of Bethlem, gave evidence that Matthews remained unhinged 'towards political subjects' and, if at large 'would be likely to be highly dangerous to the Safety of His Majesty's Person'.[34]

Matthews lost his case. This is not surprising. There was, indeed, an impressive amount of professional testimony as to his continued insanity. Moreover, George III's life had already been endangered several times by lunatics such as Margaret Nicholson and James Hadfield (themselves housed in Bethlem); no prudent court would risk a repetition, especially during a wartime crisis. And on top of all this, Haslam had been able to reveal to the court specific instructions from the Home Secretary, Lord Liverpool, requiring

Matthews's continued detention.[35] This political pressure was surely decisive.

Haslam was nettled by the whole affair, which so deeply challenged his own, and Bethlem's authority; it provoked him to write the *Illustrations*. He was perhaps above all angry at the intervention of Clutterbuck and Birkbeck. For one thing, their action seemed a breach of professional etiquette. For another, in Haslam's view, the good gentlemen were not experts in insanity – a point he made sarcastically in the *Illustrations*. Indeed the epigraph on Haslam's title page, taken from Samuel Foote, was presumably intended to apply to the pair of them ('Oh, Sir, there are in this town, Mountebanks for the mind, as well as the body!').[36] In any case, their cursory examinations could hardly be compared with the Bethlem staff's protracted experience. Above all, it struck Haslam as being a terrible scandal for medicine when doctors disagreed root-and-branch amongst themselves about the reality of mental illness.[37] If madness and reason were indeed antitheses, and if doctors reached diametrically opposite diagnoses, then one bunch of doctors must be rational and the other quite mad. The outraged Haslam did not mince his words:[38]

> Madness being the opposite to reason and good sense, as light is to darkness, straight to crooked, &c., it appears wonderful that two opposite opinions could be entertained on the subject: allowing each party to possess the ordinary faculties common to human beings in a sound and healthy state, yet such is really the fact: and if one party be right, the other must be wrong: because a person cannot correctly be said to be *in* his senses and *out* of his senses at the same time.

Haslam's hint is that Matthews was not the only person out of his mind, for he clearly felt that the dissenting doctors had been duped by their patient. Haslam's illustrations of madness thus comprise a gallery of mad doctors as well as mad patients. His polemical book (he warns readers that they may detect a sneer)[39] thus blazes away on two distinct fronts. On the one hand, he aims to demonstrate, once and for all, Matthews's madness. On the other, he seeks to vindicate the right of the Bethlem medical staff to speak authoritatively upon insanity, indeed to act as public guardians of rationality in a world which, as the opinions of 'brethren' Clutterbuck and

Introduction by Roy Porter

Birkbeck show, not all the crazy people are in the asylum. Haslam
– the man who sets himself up as the champion of medical etiquette –
is thus led into a ferocious tirade against his own profession ('it is
true, a Doctor may be blind, deaf and dumb, stupid or mad, but still
his diploma shields him from the imputation of ignorance'),[40] and
more specifically against the follies of blind dogmatists and specu-
lators, who, he hints, rather like the lunatics themselves, 'have much
practical experience, and are competent judges of all systems of
error but their own'.[41] All the same, he notes, with an explicitly
Swiftian irony, even the writings of foolish practitioners such as
Clutterbuck and Birkbeck may actually have a value, in augmenting
the 'Use and Improvement of Madness in a Commonwealth'.[42]

Believing that madness is self-incriminating, Haslam's technique is
simply to 'illustrate' it, i.e., to present it naked and verbatim to the
reader, without comment. He first offers the affidavits of Clutterbuck
and Birkbeck, testifying to Matthews's sanity – juxtaposing against
them the weightier opinion of his insanity advanced by a much
larger body of physicians (one which interestingly includes two
of the doctors who treated George III's insanity, Robert Darling
Willis and Sir Lucas Pepys, not to mention Thomas Monro, the
physician to Bethlem itself).[43] Thus the reader is invited to make up
his own mind as to which of the medical camps has reason on its side.

But then in the body of his text Haslam proceeds to 'illustrate' his
patient's madness by scrupulously and without embroidery unfold-
ing Matthews's own views. His account, he claims, is taken largely
from manuscripts of his opinions with which Matthews has been so
kind to furnish him, presumably in the parallel misguided belief that
anyone reading his views will actually be convinced of his *sanity*;
Haslam notes that words in his text placed in inverted commas are
quoted verbatim from Matthews's document. In so far as Haslam's
summaries of Matthews's views can be checked against surviving
manuscripts in Matthews's hand, his veracity and accuracy are
vindicated.[44]

Haslam chronicles how Matthews was admitted to Bethlem in
January 1797 and was transferred to the incurable establishment in
January 1798:[45]

> In this situation he continued for many years; sometimes, an
> automaton moved by the agency of persons, hereafter to be

xxxi

introduced to the notice of the reader; at others, the Emperor of the whole world, issuing proclamations to his disobedient subjects, and hurling from their thrones the usurpers of his dominions.

Having discussed the rival examinations conducted in 1809, Haslam proceeds to spell out Matthews's opinions, or in other words, his delusions.

A gang of villains, profoundly skilled in pneumatic chemistry, lives near London Wall in Moorfields, by Bethlem Hospital, and torments Matthews by means of an 'Air Loom', a diabolical machine emitting rays which possess his mind.[46] There are seven in the gang. The leader is *Bill the King*, who is most adept in working the machine. He 'has never been observed to smile'.[47] Second, there is *Jack the Schoolmaster*, who is the shorthand writer ('the recorder') to the gang.[48] Next there is *Sir Archy*, who is allegedly a woman who cross-dresses as a man, and whose language is often obscene. *Sir Archy* does not operate the mind-possessing Air Loom, but uses a magnet instead, and communicates with Matthews by the use of '*brain-sayings*', to be explained later.[49] The last of the men in the gang is the *Middle Man*; resembling the late John Smeaton the engineer, it is he who is the manufacturer of Air Looms, and thinks it all good sport.[50] Then there are three female members: *Augusta*, whose main job is to communicate with other gangs operating in the West End of London; *Charlotte*, who always speaks French, and seems to be kept no less a prisoner than Matthews is himself; and finally the *Glove Woman*, who never speaks, always wears gloves (she has the itch), and is an adept on the machine.[51] The gang hires itself out to spies, and betrays government secrets to the enemy. 'At home they lie together in promiscuous intercourse and filthy community.'[52]

The Air Loom machine which assails Matthews, works on a variety of fuels of a disgusting nature, including 'effluvia of dogs – stinking human breath – putrid effluvia – ... stench of the cesspool', and so forth.[53] Its rays assault both body and mind, producing 'a list of calamities hitherto unheard of and for which no remedy has been yet discovered'. These include '*Fluid Locking*', which renders Matthews speechless;[54] '*Cutting Soul from Sense*', which causes his feelings to be severed from his thoughts;[55] '*Stone-making*', which creates bladder stones;[56] *'Thigh-talking'*, which produces the auditory distortion of one's ear being in one's thigh;[57] *'Kiteing'*, or the capacity to hijack the brain and to implant thoughts in it beyond the control and resistance of the sufferer;[58] *'Sudden death-squeezing'* or *'Lobster-cracking'*, which involve the deployment of a magnetic field to stop the circulation and impede the vital motions;[59] *'Stomach-skinning'*, which removes the skin from the belly;[60] *'Apoplexy-working with the nutmeg grater'*, which violently forces fluids into the head, often with lethal effects;[61] *'Lengthening the brain'*, or in other words, forcible thought distortion, which can 'cause good sense to appear as insanity, and convert truth into a libel';[62] *'Thought-making'*, which is the extraction by suction of one train of thought and its replacement with another;[63] *'Laugh-making'*, which is self-explanatory; *'Poking'*, which is a form of physical punishment enforced when the victim resists the other forms of torture;[64] *'Bladder-filling'*, or implanting gas into the nerves; *'Bomb-bursting'* and *'Tying-down'*, which involve filling the whole body with a distending gas;[65] *'Gas-plucking'*, which is the extraction of the magnetic fluid from the victim's anus,[66] not to mention other tortures such as *'foot-curving, lethargy-making, spark-exploding, knee-nailing, burning-out, eye-screwing, sight-stopping, roof-stringing, vital-tearing, fibre-ripping'*, and so forth.[67]

As well as having an armoury of tortures at its disposal, the gang also mobilises various techniques of mind control. One of these is the *'brain-saying'*, which is a magnetically induced sympathetic surveillance at a distance, a silent mode of telepathic communication which Matthews first experienced when in prison in France;[68] similar to this is the *'voice-saying'*, though this involves thought control by articulate sound.[69] In his sleep Matthews is assailed by *'dream-workings'*, in which visual images are forced onto his languid mind through the medium of 'puppets' held by the gang, the images of which are impressed upon his imagination.[70] The gang is occasion-ally visible to Matthews, though they can withdraw themselves from his sight by grasping hold of a special piece of metal.[71]

Haslam then turns his attention to the Air Loom itself, of which Matthews had drawn a keyed diagram which Haslam reproduces.[72] Different levers bring the various tortures into action by producing distinct modulations of the magnetic waves, some inducing repul-sion, others attraction, some sending out metallic, others 'spermatic

animal-seminal' rays, and so forth.[73] Matthews's key explains
the workings of the different powers, for example, the 'dictating'
operations used by *Jack the Schoolmaster*.[74] Matthews (says Haslam)
believes that the Loom had been described in *Rees Cyclopaedia*,
but he assures us that no such description of course existed.[75]
Fortunately for the machine's victims, the inverse square law applies,
and the Air Loom loses its influence beyond distances of about a
thousand feet, although the bad news for lunatics is that one gang is
stationed by Bethlem and another right by St Luke's Asylum.[76]

Moreover, there are numerous gangs equipped with Air Looms at
the ready all over London, and they work the more effectively since
they employ auxiliaries ('pneumatic practitioners')[77] to pre-
magnetise people with 'volatile magnetic fluid', as they sit in coffee
houses etc,[78] to render them doubly susceptible to the action of the
Air Loom. The prime targets of the gangs – apart from Matthews
himself – are leading figures in the public administration.[79] By
injecting a minister with their rays, they can cause his mind to
become forcibly 'possessed' of a subject, or alternatively can divine
his thought processes; William Pitt himself was 'not half' susceptible.[80] As a result, such intelligence can readily be communicated to
the enemy, the French. Thus if a minister of state were thinking of
an exchange of prisoners – a topic at one stage so dear to Matthews's
heart,[81]

> the expert magnetist, having by watching and sucking, obtained
> his opinion, would immediately inform the French Minister of
> the sentiments of the English secretary, and by such means
> become enabled to baffle him in the exchange.

Such activities ('*Event-workings*', or the manipulation of happen-
ings by rays, rather in the way in which astrology was once thought
to operate)[82] were responsible for the British disasters at Walcheren
and Buenos Aires, and for the Nore Mutiny, which significantly
occurred immediately after Matthews was maliciously confined
in Bethlem, i.e., once his powers to resist the enemy had been
reduced.[83]

Matthews insists that the French had been deploying such magnetic
and mesmeric strategies right from the beginning of the war against
Britain, with a view to bringing about the 'surrendering to
the French every secret of the British Government, as for the

republicanizing Great Britain and Ireland, and particularly for dis-organizing the British navy'.[84] It was because of his own staunch resistance to these attempts that he had earlier been so persecuted by the gendarmes in Paris, and later on his return to England by the gang of seven and similar 'spy-traitor-assassins'.[85] The patriotic Matthews had disclosed all this to the Administration in 1796 through his 'incessant and loud clamours', almost daily 'writing to, or calling at the houses of, one or other of the ministers';[86] but the wily spies had succeeded in getting agents to 'pretend I was insane, for the purpose of plunging me into a madhouse, to invalidate all I said, and for the purpose of confining me within the measure of the Bedlam-attaining-airloom-warp'. Their goal had been to 'overpower my reason and speech, and destroy me in their own way, while all should suppose it was insanity which produced my death'.[87] The gangs had thus failed to silence him, but they had succeeded in having him 'forced into Bedlam'.[88] When it looked as though the celebrated lawyer, Thomas Erskine, would act as council on his behalf, they had then threatened to assail him with the rays too.[89]

Haslam unfolds in some detail the conspiracies the gangs had initiated for undermining the British war effort,[90] before drawing his account to a snappy conclusion. Matthews, he says, describes a system of 'assailment' whereby he has been deprived of volition and moral autonomy, being 'irresistibly actuated by the dextrous manoeuvres of *Bill*, or the *Middle Man*'.[91] Automata of this kind who are self-confessedly 'not responsible' for their actions 'ought not to be at large'; not least because 'already too many maniacs ... enjoy a dangerous liberty'.[92] Upon this, Haslam rests his case.

Interpretation

What is fascinating about Haslam's strategy is that he felt no need to proceed one syllable beyond his exposition of Matthews's views: he believed his patient utterly condemned himself out of his own mouth. He entertained not the slightest doubt that, *pace* Birkbeck and Clutterbuck, every right-thinking reader would conclude that Matthews was insane (a not unreasonable supposition). He felt no obligation to Matthews or to his relatives to discuss how Bethlem had handled this persecuted wretch. He did not believe it was incumbent upon him even to demonstrate in detail that Matthews was not merely deluded but was positively *dangerous* to society. He felt no obligation to psychiatric enlightenment to analyse Matthews's condition, to attempt an aetiology, to classify his delusions, or indeed to investigate their meanings. Indeed, one may surmise that for Haslam there were none; Matthews's thoughts were just the meaningless ramblings of a man gripped by delusions.[93] Haslam's work can read as a rather self-satisfied exercise, not free from a tendency to make cheap fun of a lunatic.

Unlike Haslam, we inevitably start interpreting Matthews's delusional system. It is beyond my competence to attempt a retrospective diagnosis from the standpoint of today's psychiatry, though it is clear that he would be recognized as some kind of paranoid schizophrenic.[94] Historically, it is perhaps more important to attempt to account for the content and orientation of Matthews's thought-world. Surely his experiences of being in the thick of French political machinations during the Terror, culminating in years in gaol, living in dread of the guillotine, led his imagination to an obsession with plots and persecution, intrigues, conspiracies and double-crossings. It is worth remembering that many of the most popular (and hence putatively 'rational') political ideologues of the 1790s – Edmund Burke, John Robison, the Abbé Barruel – quite explicitly interpreted the French Revolution itself as the work of subversive conspirators, and saw the Revolutionaries in turn, through further conspiracy, aiming to subvert European civilization. Official political ideology itself thus endorsed a paranoia which bears comparison with Matthews's.[95]

Next, the stage props of Matthews's system – the rays, waves and gases – directly reflected the popular sciences of the late eighteenth century. The Air Loom seems to unite public fascination with textile machinery with a concern with pneumatic chemistry ('air') as pursued by Priestley, Lavoisier, Beddoes and others.[96] Above all, the whole notion of projecting superfine aetherial waves through the atmosphere and into people, aided by magnetic powers, was directly indebted to the Mesmeric craze which had swept Paris, and to a lesser extent London, during the 1780s and 1790s. Mesmer had believed that good health, mental and physical, depended upon the free flow of such rays through the body, devising special storage machines (*baquets*) which in certain respects resembled Matthews's

Air Loom. When the flow of these waves was halted or distorted, pain, disease and death could result, in ways comparable to Matthews's *'lobster-cracking'*, *'bladder-filling'* and *'bomb-bursting'*. Whereas Mesmer had attempted to confine himself to physical cures, the Parisian Mesmerists of Matthews's time grew more interested in psychic powers – the sympathetic projection of thought and ideas at a distance – rather as in Matthews's *'brain-sayings'*.[97] It is no small irony that Matthews thus conceived of himself as being a victim of quasi-Mesmeric, thought-controlling operators, given that later dynamic psychiatrists, not least Freud, attempted to deploy Mesmeric powers for psycho-therapeutic purposes.[98]

Whatever precisely was the root cause of Matthews's malady, he clearly experienced various kinds of disturbances of, and interference with, his consciousness and body sensations. He found a language for these which attributed his inner psychic woes to, and projected them onto, external and material forces – indeed, he personified them as malign persecutors. There may be a suggestive parallel to be drawn here with the celebrated experiences of Judge Daniel Schreber approximately a century later. As his famous *Memoirs* indicate, Schreber, confined to a succession of German asylums, experienced a range of tortures upon his mind and body emanating from external persecutors. His idiosyncratic names for them – 'the compression of the chest miracle', 'the purification of the abdomen' and the 'coccyx miracle' – have patent affinities to Matthews's *'gas-plucking'*, *'bomb-bursting'* and so forth.[99] In Schreber's case we can be reasonably sure that the individual torments were literal echoes of the painful orthopaedic devices used upon him while a child by his father.[100] It is less clear whence Matthews's torments were derived; possibly from his experiences of confinement, perhaps in manacles, first in French gaols; possibly from his treatment in Bethlem itself.

It would be too literal-minded to proffer a semiotic key to each and every item in Matthews's tortured fantasy world. Nevertheless, one intriguing possibility presents itself. Who precisely were the gang of seven operating around the environs of Bethlem? Were they not, in fact, the staff, the doctors, attendants, or indeed the patients, of Bethlem itself? (Let us not forget that Matthews tells us that a similar gang operated at St Luke's.) Such characters would clearly have it in their power to inject the thought disturbance commonly called 'brain-sayings' into the heads of the inmates; they would certainly have been able to read their minds (after all, that form of spying is precisely what Haslam had undertaken with Matthews: do we here see the model for *Jack the Schoolmaster*, who records all?).[101] Not least, they would have had unlimited 'torturing' powers at their disposal; after all, the 1815 Commons inquiry found mechanical restraints such as irons and fetters still widespread at Bethlem, and apparently used as punishments.[102] It would be an exquisite irony if Matthews has cast the staff of Bethlem, including Haslam himself, as the *dramatis personae* in his fantasy world of persecutors; and if Haslam has solemnly recorded it (as the deluded symptoms of a madman!) without the least inkling that it might actually apply to himself, indeed be the indictment of himself as a torturer. Haslam described Matthews in print. But in doing so, he perhaps also, quite unwittingly, described Matthews describing Haslam. Self-incriminatingly, like Dogberry, he has himself written down an ass.

Aftermath

Haslam won the battle but not the war. Matthews remained within Bethlem. He was a rather unusual patient. He had learnt calligraphy and technical drawing and when a public competition was announced for designs for the new Bethlem building, Matthews drew up a forty-six page dossier of architectural designs (now lost), which the governors so commended that they voted him an *ex gratia* payment of £30. Allegedly 'for a change of air', to improve his ailing health, he was moved (as it were on parole) in 1814 to Fox's London House asylum at Hackney (half the fees were paid by Bethlem, half by his relatives), where he made himself useful as 'advising manager' on the patients, a nice instance of poacher turned gamekeeper.[103] His relatives made further requests for his release, but once again government pressure, stressing that Matthews had been designated a dangerous lunatic, proved decisive.[104] He died there in 1815. From the grave, however, he had the last laugh on Haslam.

The House of Commons committee of 1815 brought up the Matthews case once more, to Haslam's embarrassment. It was alleged by a nephew of Matthews, Richard Staveley, a wholesale druggist, that Matthews had been set in leg locks by Haslam for challenging his 'authority', and had been chained up as a punishment to 'let you know what our authority is'. According to Staveley, Matthews was recognized by most staff and patients alike to be a harmless person – a peacemaker even – who had had the misfortune to incur Haslam's 'violent animosity'. Haslam's involvement in the refusal to allow Matthews's release was made to look like sheer cussedness. It is hard in retrospect to tell precisely how dangerous Haslam really believed Matthews to be, or whether he primarily felt compelled to act under political orders from the government.[105]

In the ensuing witchhunt to find a scapegoat for the scandalous revelations, the Bethlem governors apparently had access to a document written by Matthews, accusing Haslam of malpractice. It appears that Matthews had earlier threatened to make this document public, in fact (so Haslam noted) 'pluming himself on the retaliation he could make for the supposed injuries he had received, he read to me the greater part of it'. Haslam twice printed defences of his conduct, complaining *inter alia* that the governors themselves had been fooled by Matthews's false accusations:[106]

> I conceived that its circulation ought not to be prevented, on the presumption that there existed in the judgment of those who passed for persons of sound mind, a sufficient disrelish for absurdity, to enable them to discriminate the transactions of daylight, from the materials of a dream.

Haslam's defence of his actions hardly tried to conceal the scandalous condition of Bethlem (the surgeon a drunken madman, the matron a slut, the keepers pilferers, etc.), instead shuffling off his own responsibility for the disgrace. Unimpressed, the governors dismissed him in 1816. He saw himself as 'sacrificed to public clamour and party spirit' – a phrase ironically echoing Matthews's lamentations! At the age of fifty-two, he found himself without post or a pension.

An energetic man, Haslam set about putting himself back on his feet. He sold his library, bought an MD from Marischal College, Aberdeen, and set up as a physician, being admitted a Licentiate of the Royal College of Physicians in 1824 at the ripe old age of sixty. To supplement his income he penned numerous psychiatric works, and droll pieces for the *Literary Gazette* besides.[107] He survived till

1844. His perception of the rampancy of madness increased with age. Appearing as a forensic witness in one court case he was asked if the defendant were of sound mind. 'I never saw any human being', he replied, 'who was of sound mind'. When counsel objected that this was no proper answer, Haslam added, 'I presume the Deity is of sound mind, and He alone'. Asked how he knew this, Haslam answered 'from my own reflections during the last fourteen years, and from repeated conversations with the best divines in the country'.[108]

The history of psychiatry is the saga of infinitely complicated interactions between patients and psychiatrists.[109] Both parties have described the other, in terms generally not the most flattering. Each has attempted to exercise control over the other – in the case of the mad, by means that have to be devious. Operating within each other's field of force, they readily become doubles. The duel between John Haslam and James Tilly Matthews forms a complex and intriguing example of this *folie à deux*.

Notes

1. M. Roth and J. Kroll (1986) *The Reality of Mental Illness*, Cambridge: Cambridge University Press; for a different defence of a comparable position see P. Sedgwick (1982) *Psycho Politics*, London: Pluto Press.
2. For this view see M. MacDonald (1981) *Mystical Bedlam: Madness, Anxiety and Healing in Seventeenth Century England*, Cambridge: Cambridge University Press; Roy Porter (1987) *Mind Forg'd Manacles. A history of madness in England from the Restoration to the Regency*, London: Athlone Press, pp. 33–40.
3. See G. Becker (1978) *The Mad Genius Controversy*, Beverly Hills: Sage; M. Screech (1980) *Ecstasy and the Praise of Folly*, London: Duckworth, and 'Good Madness in Christendom', in W. F. Bynum, Roy Porter and Michael Shepherd (eds) (1985) *The Anatomy of Madness*, London: Tavistock, 2 vols, 1: 25–39.
4. E. G. O'Donoghue (1914) *The Story of Bethlem Hospital from its Foundation in 1247*, London: Fisher & Unwin; A. Masters (1972) *Bedlam*, London: Michael Joseph; S. Gilman (1982) *Seeing the Insane*, New York: Brunner, Mazel.
5. T. Szasz (1972) *The Manufacture of Madness*, London: Paladin; Szasz (1972) *The Myth of Mental Illness*, London: Granada; Szasz

(1975) *The Age of Madness. The History of Involuntary Hospitalization Presented in Selected Texts*, London: Routledge & Kegan Paul. For recent evaluation see Joan Busfield (1986) *Managing Madness. Changing Ideas and Practice*, London: Hutchinson.

6. Porter, op. cit. (note 2), ch. 3; for a contrary view see M. Foucault (1965) *Madness and Civilization. A History of Insanity in the Age of Reason*, A. Sheridan (trans.), New York: Random House.

7. A. Scull (1979) *Museums of Madness*, London: Allen Lane.

8. See generally T. Butler (1985) *Mental Health, Social Policy and the Law*, London: Macmillan; K. Jones (1955) *Lunacy, Law and Conscience, 1744–1845*, London: Routledge & Kegan Paul.

8a. Alexander Cruden (1739) *The London Citizen Exceedingly Injured*, London.

9. W. Parry-Jones (1972) *The Trade in Lunacy, A Study of Private Madhouses in England in the Eighteenth and Nineteenth Centuries*, London: Routledge & Kegan Paul; Porter, op. cit. (note 2), ch. 3.

9a. Samuel Bruckshaw (1774) *The Case, Petition and Address of Samuel Bruckshaw, who suffered a Most Severe Imprisonment for Very Near the Whole Year ...*, London.

9b. Samuel Bruckshaw (1774) *One More Proof of the Iniquitous Abuse of Private Madhouses*, London.

10. See the discussion in D. A. Peterson (1982) *A Mad People's History of Madness*, Pittsburgh: University of Pittsburgh Press.

11. P. McCandless (1981) 'Liberty and Lunacy: The Victorians and Wrongful Confinement', in Andrew Scull (ed.) *Madhouses, Mad Doctors and Madmen*, London: Athlone Press, pp. 253–74.

12. Porter, op. cit. (note 2), pp. 165–8.

13. J. Parkinson (1811) *Mad-houses. Observations on the Act for Regulation of Mad-Houses and A Correction of the Statements of the Case of Benjamin Elliott, Convicted of Illegally Confining Mary Daintree: With Remarks Addressed to the Friends of Insane Persons*, London: Sherwood, Neeley and Jones.

14. These issues are discussed in the first two chapters of Roy Porter (1987) *A Social History of Madness*, London: Weidenfeld & Nicolson.

15. Parliamentary Papers (1815) *Report (4) from the Committee on Madhouses in England*, House of Commons.

16. For information on Matthews see Roy Porter (1985) '"Under the Influence": Mesmerism in England', *History Today*, September: 22–9; David Williams (1980) *Incidents in my own Life which have been Thought of Some Importance*, Peter France (ed.), Falmer: University of Sussex Library, pp. 10, 28, 32–4, 60; D. Williams (1938) 'The Missions of David Williams and James Tilly Matthews to

England (1793)', *English Historical Review*, 53: 651–68 (an excellent article, based upon unpublished documents in the French archives); D. Williams (1938) 'Un document inédit sur la Gironde', *Annales historiques de la Révolution française*, xv: 430–1; J. G. Alger (1889) *Englishmen in the French Revolution*, London; Sampson, Low & Co. Contemporaries often spelt Matthews's middle name 'Tilley' but he signed himself 'Tilly'.

17. France (ed.), op. cit. (note 16), p. 33. David Williams (1736–1816) was a man of letters and a political libertarian. He visited France in 1792, becoming a French citizen, and remaining till the execution of Louis XVI, which he deplored. He was involved in peace negotiations with Lord Grenville (William Wyndham, 1759–1834), at this time Secretary of State for Foreign Affairs.

18. British Library, Add. MS. 38231, fo.82. Charles Jenkinson (1727–1808) had been elevated first Earl of Liverpool in 1796. He was a veteran of Lord North's administrations, serving under Pitt, and becoming Chancellor of the Duchy of Lancaster. He was deeply involved in the mid 1790s in negotiations with the Dutch and the French.

19. British Library, MS. 38231, fo.121. There is one further letter of Matthews to Liverpool (Add. MS. 38231, fo.125). Addressed from Camberwell Grove and dated 24 December 1796 it runs:

> My Lord,
> Having left with the Right Hon. Earl Moira a Narrative of Facts which I have experienced, I beg to refer your Lordship to that Independent Nobleman for their Perusal, as your Lordships name is therein mentioned. I have the honour to be my Lord I am your Lordships mo. Obt. Servant, James Tilly Matthews.

Lord Moira (Francis Hastings: 1754–1826) was a soldier in command of various expeditionary forces in the mid 1790s.

20. John Haslam (1810) *Illustrations of Madness, Exhibiting a Singular Case of Insanity, and a No Less Remarkable Difference of Medical Opinion: Developing the Nature of Assailment, and the Manner of Working Events; with a Description of the Tortures Experienced by Bomb-Bursting, Lobster-Cracking and Lengthening the Brain, Embellished with a Curious Plate*, London: Rivingtons, Robinsons, Callow, Murray & Greenland, p. 1; Porter (1985), op. cit. (note 16); Williams (1980), op. cit. (note 16), p. 34. These proceedings are extensively documented in the Governors' Minute Books for the period, at the Bethlem Archives.

21. Ibid., p. 2.

22. For biographical information see Richard Hunter and Ida Macalpine (1962) 'John Haslam: His Will and his Daughter', *Medical History*, 6: 22–6; D. Leigh (1955) 'John Haslam, M.D. 1764–1844', *Journal of the History of Medicine*, 10: 17–43, and Leigh (1961) *The Historical Development of British Psychiatry*, Oxford: Pergamon, vol. 1. It is unfortunate that Leigh persistently refers to *John* Tilly Matthews, whom he labels a 'formidable trouble-maker' (p. 110).

23. Bryan Crowther (1811) *Practical Remarks on Insanity*, London: Thomas Underwood.

24. Parliamentary Papers (1815), op. cit. (note 15), p. 104.

25. A. Scull, op. cit. (note 7), pp. 76f.; Parliamentary Papers (1815), op. cit. (note 15), pp. 63f., 82f.

26. See the discussion in Leigh (1961) *Development of British Psychiatry*, op. cit. (note 22), pp. 110–11; O'Donoghue (1914), op. cit. (note 4), pp. 272ff.

27. There is a sensible discussion in Leigh (1961) *Development of British Psychiatry*, op. cit. (note 22), pp. 116–17, 136; Leigh believes Haslam did indeed offer a clear and accurate clinical description of *dementia praecox*. Leigh regards Haslam as the leading European psychiatrist of his age, placing him, for example, above Pinel: p. 144. However highly one judges Haslam's practical common sense, this view is distinctly eccentric.

28. J. Haslam (1817) *Medical Jurisprudence, as it Relates to Insanity, According to the Law of England*, London: R. Hunter, quoted in Leigh (1961) *Development of Psychiatry*, op. cit. (note 22), p. 128. See also D. Leigh (1954) 'John Haslam, M.D., A Pioneer of Forensic Psychiatry', *British Journal of Delinquency*, 4: 201–6.

29. J. Haslam (1809) *Observations on Madness and Melancholy, including Practical Remarks on those Diseases; Together with Cases: and an Account of the Morbid Appearance on Dissection*, 2nd edn, considerably enlarged, London: J. Callow, quoted in Leigh (1961) *Development of British Psychiatry*, op. cit. (note 22), p. 121.

30. See Porter (1987) op. cit. (note 2), pp. 209–28; Leigh (1961) *Development of British Psychiatry*, op. cit. (note 22), p. 122. For Haslam 'moral management' did not preclude physical restraint.

31. This is documented in Haslam (1810) *Illustrations of Madness* (note 22), pp. 4f. According to the testimony of Richard Staveley, Matthews's nephew, before the 1815 Parliamentary committee, Clutterbuck found Matthews disturbed on only one point, the Air Loom. Since this was merely 'philosophical', it was harmless: p. 14. Henry Clutterbuck was a licentiate of the Royal College of Physicians, and one of the physicians to the General Dispensary. He was author of a

number of medical treatises including (1819) *Observations on the Prevention and Treatment of the Epidemic Fever at Present Prevailing in this Metropolis and Most Parts of the United Kingdom*, London: Longman, Rees, Orme & Brown. George Birkbeck (1776–1841) had graduated MD at Edinburgh in 1796 and, after serving as professor of natural philosophy at the Andersonian Institution in Glasgow, set up as a physician in London, becoming a licentiate of the Royal College of Physicians in 1808. He is chiefly remembered as a founder of the Mechanics' Institute movement. See also H. Clutterbuck (1842) *A Brief Memoir of George Birkbeck, M.D.*, London: the Medical Society of London. Birkbeck and Clutterbuck were both physicians to the General Dispensary in Aldersgate Street.

32. See deposition of Robert Dunbar (29 November 1809), Bethlem Archives, Box 61(8).

33. See deposition of John Haslam (30 November 1809), Bethlem Archives, Box 61 (8). This is reproduced in full below in Appendix 2.

34. See deposition of Richard Baldwyn (2 December 1809), Bethlem Archives, Box 61(8).

35. See Bethlem Archives, Box 61(8).

36. Haslam (1810) *Illustrations of Madness*, op. cit. (note 20), p. 19 ('the practice of the two doctors shall be left to the humane construction of the Christian reader').

37. Ibid., p. 16.

38. Ibid., p. 15.

39. Ibid., p. vi.

40. Ibid., p. 16.

41. Ibid., p. 18.

42. Ibid., p. vi. Haslam's allusion is of course to the 'Digression' in Swift's *Tale of a Tub*.

43. Ibid., p. 15. Haslam affirmed Matthews's insanity before the Parliamentary Committee: Parliamentary Papers (1815) op. cit. (note 15), pp. 90f. Haslam claimed that he had seen Matthews 'violent'. He also stated that he had had Matthews taught the art of engraving.

44. In the Archives of the Royal Bethlem Hospital there is a manuscript of Matthews's, which confirms to Haslam's view that Matthews thought of himself as a world emperor. This manuscript is reproduced as Appendix 3.

45. Haslam (1810) *Illustrations of Madness*, op. cit. (note 20), p. 2.

46. Ibid., p. 19.

47. Ibid., p. 21.

48. Ibid., p. 22.

49. Ibid., p. 23.

50. Ibid., p. 24.
51. Ibid., pp. 25–7.
52. Ibid., p. 21.
53. Ibid., p. 28.
54. Ibid., p. 30.
55. Ibid., p. 30.
56. Ibid., p. 30.
57. Ibid., p. 31.
58. Ibid., pp. 31–2.
59. Ibid., p. 33.
60. Ibid., p. 33.
61. Ibid., p. 33.
62. Ibid., p. 34.
63. Ibid., pp. 34–5.
64. Ibid., pp. 35–6.
65. Ibid., p. 36.
66. Ibid., pp. 37–8.
67. Ibid., p. 38.
68. Ibid., pp. 38–9.
69. Ibid., p. 40.
70. Ibid., pp. 40–1.
71. Ibid., pp. 41–2.
72. Ibid., pp. 42–9.
73. Ibid., p. 49.
74. Ibid., p. 50.
75. Ibid., p. 45.
76. Ibid., p. 51.
77. Ibid., p. 53.
78. Ibid., p. 53.
79. Ibid., p. 54.
80. Ibid., p. 68.
81. Ibid., p. 55.
82. Ibid., p. 60.
83. Ibid., p. 64.
84. Ibid., p. 61.
85. Ibid., p. 63.
86. Ibid., p. 64.
87. Ibid., p. 64.
88. Ibid., p. 66.
89. Ibid., p. 73.
90. Ibid., p. 70.
91. Ibid., p. 80.

92. Ibid., p. 80.
93. For the history of the development of that aspect of psychiatry which denies meanings to madness, see Porter (1987) *Social History of Madness*, op. cit. (note 14), ch. 2.
94. He has been called a 'a clear paranoid' by M. D. Altschule (1977) *Origins of Concepts in Human Behavior*, New York: Halstead Press, ch. 6., and as having 'Schneiderian First Rank Symptoms' by Peter Carpenter (1987) 'Schizophrenia 1810 – James Tilly Matthews and the Air Loom', unpublished paper, and a schizophrenic in J. E. Meyer and Ruth Meyer (1969) 'Selbstzeugnisse eines Schizophrenen um 1800', *Confinia Psychiatrica*, 12: 130–43; Leigh (1961) *Development of British Psychiatry*, op. cit. (note 22), says he was suffering from 'paranoid Schizophrenia', p. 109. No Freudian has yet, it seems, decoded Matthews's paranoia, which, according to normal Freudian interpretations, would be expected to be symptomatic of repressed homosexual desires (? towards Haslam). The intrepid Freudian could find material in Matthews's testimony upon which to work, not least the transvestite *Sir Archy*, and Matthews's habit of calling allied foreign troops 'Mollys', slang for homosexuals.
95. For these points made in greater detail see Porter (1987) *Mind Forg'd Manacles*, op. cit. (note 2), pp. 233–4, 243–4, and I. Kramnick (1977) *The Rage of Edmund Burke*, New York: Basic Books.
96. For fascination with machines see H. Jennings (1985) *Pandaemonium*, London: André Deutsch.
97. See Darnton (1968) *Mesmerism and the End of the Enlightenment in France*, Cambridge, Mass.: Harvard University Press. G. Sutton (1981) 'Electric Medicine and Mesmerism', *Isis*, 72: 375–92; V. Buranelli (1975) *The Wizard from Vienna*, New York: Peter Owen; J. Miller, 'Mesmerism', *The Listener* (22 November 1973); Williams (1938), op. cit. (note 16).
98. H. F. Ellenberger (1971) *The Discovery of the Unconscious: The History and Evolution of Dynamic Psychiatry*, New York: Basic Books.
99. D. P. Schreber, *Memoirs of My Nervous Illness*, by Ida Macalpine and R. Hunter (trans and eds) (1955), London: William Dawson & Sons.
100. M. Schatzman (1973) *Soul Murder: Persecution in the Family*, London: Allen Lane.
101. Haslam (1810) *Illustrations of Madness*, op. cit. (note 20), p. 22.
102. *Parliamentary Papers* (1815), op. cit. (note 15), pp. 92f.
103. For these details see Leigh (1961) *Development of British Psychiatry* op. cit. (note 22), pp. 134f. Dr John Coakley Lettsom, a Camberwell

neighbour, testified to Matthews's ailing health. See Bethlem Archives, Governors' Minute Book, 11 August 1814. It is noteworthy that Dr Samuel Fox did not believe Matthews insane. This suggests that it was confinement specifically in Bethlem which triggered his condition.

104. See Bethlem Archives, Governors' Minute Book, 11 August 1814, letter from Lord Sidmouth, who was Home Secretary.
105. Parliamentary Papers (1815), op. cit. (note 15), pp. 14–16. The unspoken assumption behind the evidence about Matthews presented to the Commons committee was that the Bethlem medical staff were unwilling to have Matthews released lest he spilt the beans about the inhumane conditions obtaining there.
106. Leigh (1961) *Development of British Psychiatry*, op. cit. (note 22), p. 132; J. Haslam (1819) *A Letter to the Governors of Bethlem Hospital*, London: Taylor & Hessey.
107. Leigh (1961) *Development of British Psychiatry*, op. cit. (note 22), pp. 139f.; F. Schiller (1984) 'Haslam of "Bedlam", Kitchiner of the "Oracles": Two Doctors under their Mad King George III, and their Friendship', *Medical History*, 28: 189–201.
108. Quoted in N. Walker (1968) *Crime and Insanity in England*, Edinburgh: Edinburgh University Press, 1: 89.
109. For discussion see Porter (1987) *Social History of Madness*, op. cit. (note 14), ch. 2; P. Barham (1984) *Schizophrenia and Human Values*, Oxford: Basil Blackwell.

APPENDIX 1

Bibliography of the Writings of John Haslam

J. Haslam (1798) *Observations on Insanity, with Practical Remarks on the Disease and an Account of the Morbid Appearance on Dissection*, London: F. & C. Rivington.

J. Haslam (1809) *Observations on Madness and Melancholy, including Practical Remarks on those Diseases; together with Cases: and an Account of the Morbid Appearances on Dissection*, 2nd edn, considerably enlarged, London: J. Callow.

J. Haslam (1810) *Illustrations of Madness: Exhibiting a Singular Case of Insanity, and No Less Remarkable Difference of Medical Opinion: Developing the Nature of Assailment, and the Manner of Working Events; with a Description of the Tortures Experienced by Bomb-Bursting, Lobster-Cracking, and Lengthening the Brain, Embellished with a Curious Plate*, London: Rivingtons, Robinsons, Callow, Murray & Greenland.

J. Haslam (1816) *Observations of the Physician and Apothecary of Bethlem Hospital, upon the Evidence Taken Before the Committee of the Hon. House of Commons for Regulating Mad-Houses*, London: H. Bryer.

J. Haslam (1817) *Considerations on the Moral Management of Insane Persons*, London: R. Hunter.

J. Haslam (1817) *Medical Jurisprudence, as it Relates to Insanity, According to the Law of England*, London: R. Hunter.

J. Haslam (1818) *A Letter to the Governors of Bethlem Hospital, Containing an Account of their Management of that Institution for the Last Twenty Years; Elucidated by Original Letters and Authentic Documents; with a Correct Narrative of the Confinement of James Norris, by Order of their Subcommittee; and Interesting Observations on the Parliamentary Proceedings*, London: Taylor & Hessey.

J. Haslam (1819) *Sound Mind; or, Contributions to the Natural History and Physiology of the Human Intellect*, London: Longman, Hurst, Rees, Orme & Brown.

J. Haslam (1823) *A Letter to the Right Honourable, the Lord Chancellor, on the Nature and Interpretation of Unsoundness of Mind, and Imbecility of Intellect*, London: R. Hunter.

J. Haslam (1827–8) 'Lectures on the Intellectual Composition of Man', *The Lancet*, 1: 38, 71, 119, 207, 288, 335.

J. Haslam (1835) *On the Nature of Thought, or the Act of Thinking, and its Connexion with a Perspicuous Sentence*, London: Longman, Rees, Orme, Brown, Greene & Longman.

J. Haslam (1850) *Selection of Papers and Prize Essays on Subjects Connected with Insanity*, Read Before the Society for Improving the Conditions of the Insane, London: published by the Society.

APPENDIX 2

Deposition of James Haslam before King's Bench November 1809

In the Kings Bench

John Haslam the Apothecary of Bethlem Hospital maketh oath and saith that he has been upwards of 25 years engaged in the profession of medicine during which time his attention has been principally directed to the cure and treatment of mental diseases that during such time he has had the examination of several thousand Patients and from his particular situation at Bethlem Hospital for the last 14 years or thereabouts has had the most constant opportunities of studying this disease in all its forms.

And this Deponent saith that he has been acquainted with the case of the Patient James Tilley Matthews from the time of his first coming into the Hospital which was on the 28th January 1797 down to the present period, and that it is his decided opinion, as it has ever been, that such Patient is a person of insane and disordered mind and that his insanity is of a tendency so dangerous to his Majesty and his Family in the particular as to the Judicature and Magistracy of the Country in general that it would be highly unsafe for him to be at large until he be sufficiently recovered to perceive the incongruity of his former opinions and to show that his renunciation of them is sincere.

And this Deponent in confirmation of the above statement further saith that at the time of the Patient first coming into the Hospital the Parish of Camberwell were his securities who were either induced or obliged by the Magistrates of Bow Street to enter into the usual Bond for him. From the notes of his case taken at that period by this Deponent it appears that 3 months before that time he had cried out Treason in the House of Commons at the time the House was sitting and his own account of himself to this Deponent at his admission was that he had been employed by the French and English Governments to negotiate a

1

peace but that he had never received any reward, not even his travelling expences. That he had been Four times backwards and forwards from France to England. That at his suggestion of its propriety, the Committee of Public Safety in France was formed and that it was in order to prevent his letters from reaching France and himself from going over there that the Traitorous Correspondence Bill in this country was received. That when he communicated to the Ministry of this Country some valuable and important secrets they betrayed him, and when he afterwards went to Paris he was there told he was betrayed and that his ruin was endeavoured to be accomplished. That they sought out in all the Provinces of France for persons of the names of Pitt and Grenville who were brought forward to claim acquaintance with him in order to destroy him. That when he was in Flanders the Duke of York caused his army to make various marches and countermarches to beset him, and wished to deliver him over to the Enemy as a spy. That the report of the Jewels of the Queen of France being stolen was a deception. They were sent over to this country as a bribe to some of the Royal Family to betray this nation and to dismember Scotland and Ireland from this Country. That the King of Prussia was at the bottom of a deception scheme by which the Duke of York was to have been made King of France and that the Princesses of this country were to have intermarried with some of the Emigrant Princes. That the King of Prussia also had formed a plan of destroying General Washington and to have divided America into two Monarchies which were to have been ruled by two of the younger Princes of this country, and that the discovery of this scheme was the cause of the late resignation of the Presidentship of the United States. That he (Matthews) hoped he should live and that he would never rest until he had brought some people in administration and also some of the Royal Family to the Block, and that when he called out Treason in the House of Commons they durst not arrest him lest he should discover the authors of the Plot.

And this Deponent further saith that he is enabled to state from his Note book that on the 10th March following his admission, he the said Matthews came down to the gate and said there was a conspiracy to destroy his Wife and Family, and that this Deponent was under the direction and influence of the Duke of Portland to detain him in the Hospital and that he would be revenged on this Deponent for detaining him there unjustly and that the water of the Pump was poisoned.

And this Deponent saith (having refreshed his memory from his said Note Book of that period) that the said Patient on the 11th March said that his being under confinement was only a part of a grand conspiracy to deprive him of his liberty which had for many years been attempted in the different Courts of Europe that he was determined to prosecute the

Hospital, the Committee this Deponent. He further said that whenever he went out there were persons before and behind him to watch where he went and that those people were employed by one of the Secretaries to Mr Pitt. That his being detained in the Hospital was to prevent his impeaching some of the Ministers of this Country and some of our Royal Family of High Treason. That Lord Mansfield, the Marquis of Bath and the Empress of Russia died of poison.

And this Deponent further saith that on the 14th April then following the Patient refused to associate with any of the said Patients in the Hospital alledging as his reason that he conceived them not to be mad, but instruments of intrigue who were paid by certain Agents to counterfeit the disease.

And this Deponent saith that the persons so alledged by the said Matthews to be hired as agents for the purpose of deception were not persons of that description but were actually insane Patients in the Hospital for medical treatment and cure. And the said Matthews further said that he believed certain pains in his joints had been produced by medicine as drugs secretly conveyed into his food and he suspected there was going on certain chemical or magnetical influence in the Hospital to his prejudice. In the August following when the Patient's Brother came to Matthews he (Matthews) said that some intrigue had forced him his Brother up to town to destroy his (the said Matthews) happiness and ruin him, although the said brother came from Birmingham with another Patient as this Deponent has been informed and believes.

And this Deponent saith that on the 10th January 1798 the Patient said there was the figure of a man on the top of Bloomsbury Church who had got a Book under his Arm. That it was Doomsday book, and that no one could open that book but himself the said Matthews. And that from the moment he the said Matthews came into the Hospital the whole of its revenues became his property.

And this Deponent further saith that after the said patient had continued in the Hospital a year, the usual period of probation, he was upon examination and consideration of his case by the proper medical officers and Committee declared a fit object to continue in the House as an incurable: Patient and more particularly from his madness having assumed the most marked features of hostility and vengeance to their Majesties and many branches of the Royal Family from his having accused the persons in power of treasonable practices from his contempt of all constituted authorities together with threats of personal revenge to the Governors Officers of Bethlem Hospital.

And this Deponent saith that in or about the year 1800, as nearly as to the time as this Deponent is able to speak from recollection, the said

Matthews was brought up before the late Lord Kenyon the Lord Chief Justice of the Court of Kings Bench at his Lordships house in Lincolns Inn Fields where he was attended by the Physician, by this Deponent and the Porter of the Hospital and that after a short intercession in which his Lordship was fully convinced of the Insanity of the Patient (he having insisted before Lord Kenyon that the Queen of England had for treasonable purposes become possessed of the Jewels of the Queen of France) he was upon the said conviction of his Lordship as to his Insanity remanded to Bethlem Hospital.

And this Deponent saith that after this period his derangement of mind became more systematic and embraced a greater variety of objects. He conceived himself to be the Emperor of the whole world and that the reigning Sovereigns, were Impostors and Usurpers and more, particularly directed his threats towards his present Majesty and the Royal Family deriving his own right to the Crown from King Edward the 3rd. And there is in this Deponent's possession a very large quantity of documents in the hand writing of the said Patient which are very voluminous and to which it is therefore impossible to do more than refer – but which are open to inspection and contain the most solemn assertions of his own titles and dignities being paramount to all [illeg.] and denouncing vengeance and death against his Majesty, the Members of the Divine Council, Secretaries of State, Judges, Governors of the Hospital and all other authorities offering different rewards for their lives and complaining of the most tyrannical, illegal and cruel treatment.

And this Deponent further saith that after the period of his return from the examination by Lord Kenyon the Patients told this Deponent that a magnet was placed in the centre of his brain by which a number of event workers and political chemists were enabled to attain his thoughts and persisted that these persons he said he constantly heard. They forced him to utter various noises and had the power of directing his thoughts; they also endeavoured to poison him by admitting into his room various stenches – From this period until the applications which have been made within the last year or two by his friends, the patient has on examination unequivocally shown abundant proofs of insanity to this Deponent and as this Deponent believes to all such medical persons as have occasionally examined him but for about the said period of a year or two past the said patient appears to have been aware that his particular hallucination or weak part was Politics and that when he has been interrogated upon the subjects of his former opinions he has generally replied that he should give no answer to such questions that he had firmly resolved never to commit himself upon the subject of Politics, and that whatever attempts might be made no power on earth should ever induce him to advert to the subject again, but this Deponent saith that when he has been asked whether he renounced any of those opinions formerly held by him he has declared that he remained of the same opinions and never would renounce them – when he has been asked whether he was ever insane, he has always declared that he never was insane at any period of his life but always in his perfect senses and that his whole confinement in the hospital has been an injust imprisonment without having for its real cause that which had been always assigned, namely.

And this Deponent further saith that he apprehends as a medical question he is well warranted in putting the question of his sanity or insanity upon such issue and in stating that the Patient is not now of sound mind or he could have no objection to converse or be questioned upon those subjects where he is well aware his derangement would be manifest.

And this Deponent further saith that so far from having been able to obtain from the Patient a renunciation of his former errors he never would confess that he was at any time under the influence of an unsound judgment under which in this Deponent's opinion he still remains and which is among the reasons of the Patient's not being able to satisfy such persons as have been more particularly accustomed to the treatment of mental disease of his being in a sound state of mind.

And this Deponent saith that within the space of the last week the said Patient has declared in the presence and hearing of this Deponent and of the various Physicians who have examined him (in addition to many said proofs of lunacy exhibited at the same time) that there had long been and was then an immense Machine under ground near the Hospital under the management of powerful and evil agents with whom he the said Matthews had frequently had intercourse by means of which Machine he the said Matthews was acted upon and impregnated to his great and serious injury, and that many other persons were likewise under such malignant influence and that the infallible proofs of such agency being exerted upon any particular persons was that at the time of such persons swallowing, a noise was heard by them like the creaking of a wicker basket when pressed together.

And this Deponent further saith that with respect to the conversation stated in the Affidavit of Mr Robert Dunbar to have taken place with this Deponent in a Coffee House he this Deponent never to his knowledge or belief saw the said Mr Dunbar in any Coffee House or a place of meeting nor ever conversed with him upon any subject until the said Mr Dunbar appeared at the Hospital a few months since and charged this Deponent with using such words and that the expressions so referred to him this Deponent assuredly be the consequence of inaccuracy or misconception

on the part of the said Mr Dunbar inasmuch as this Deponent's opinion
has always remained unaltered upon the subject of the said Patient's
continued lunacy and is well known to have so remained.
Sworn at my Chambers Sergeants from Chancery Lane the 1st day of
December 1809.
Before me. J. Bayley

John Haslam

Haslam also circulated a letter from Lord Liverpool's office:

Whitehall 7th September
1809

Gentlemen,
   I recommend that you do continue to detain in your Hospital as a fit
and proper subject James Tilley Matthews a lunatic who is at present
under your charge, and care shall be taken that the customary expenses of
cloathing etc together with the Expenses of his funeral in case he dies
there shall be defrayed

I have the honour to be
Gentlemen your most obedient
humble servant (signed)
Liverpool

To the Right Worshipful the President and Treasurer and the Worshipful
the Governors of Bethlem Hospital.

Haslam continued:

If this letter had not been sent Governors would not have felt themselves
justified in preventing the Patient's discharge but considering they themselves to be acting in perfect safety under the conviction of his complete
madness and under the further sanction of such Letter they have detained
him till now – the only object has been the public security and they can
have now no other – In every other view it is highly desirable to them
that he should be discharged, but it will remain to be seen what sort of
security the Friends are prepared to give to the Court and country for the
safe custody of a man who upon the above Affidavits will it is presumed
be proved insane – The Committee have paused because no assurance has
ever been given them on which they could rely that the Patient should be
confined. On the contrary the applicants have always declared they
believed him sane and therefore it could not be expected they should

provide for his custody – They still remain of the same opinion with regard to his sanity of the fallacy of which it would perhaps be impossible for any weight of Evidence to convince them.

With respect to the letter of Lord Liverpool – it has hitherto been judged advisable on the part of the Hospital to give it no prominence on the present occasion but as it is sworn by one of the Patient's friends that he has been informed by one of the Hospital Committee that there is such a Letter, and as the Judge is very likely to make some enquiries on that head, a few words on the reason of its being sent have been already said. The Patient first came in it is true from the parish of Camberwell but that parish was Ordered if not compelled by the Magistrates of Bow Street to send the Patient to the Hospital. At that time the Act of Parliament authorizing the confinement of Lunatic troublesome to the King was not passed and therefore no official Letter could then be sent. The Patient however was always considered as in the Hospital by the Order and with the knowledge of Government and when it appeared to the Governors that they were no longer justified in detaining him except under the written authority of Government they judged it advisable at all events that the Government should be informed of his continued insanity and of the pressing applications that were not withstanding made for his discharge leaving it to themselves to act in the matter or not as they should see fit. The Letter therefore was sent upon such information.

It is most probable that it will not be deemed advisable to notice the information so communicated to Government however honourable the motives by which the governors were really actuated.

If the Judge shall now be satisfied that he ought to discharge the Patient the Governors will be perfectly satisfied; also far from having any Interest in his detention their very constitution as one of charity renders it their obvious interest to keep the number of such unhappy Persons as low as possible; and the very great and most improper trouble occasioned for many years past both to the Governors and Officers by the detention of this particular Patient renders his discharge truly desirable. The Governors however are not unmindful that they have a serious duty to perform by the Sovereign and the Public as well as by the Patients and their friends and they have therefore pursued the line of conduct which the above Affidavits will explain and (it is hoped) will justify.

APPENDIX 3

Writing by James Tilly Matthews, probably intended to be used by Haslam as evidence in the King's Bench case

James, Absolute, Sole, & Supreme Sacred Omni Imperious Arch Grand Arch Sovereign Omni Imperious Arch Grand Arch Proprietor Omni Imperious Arch-Grand-Arch-Emperor-Supreme etc. March the Twentieth One Thousand Eight hundred & four

The following are the Rewards by Me offered so long ago Issued for the putting to Death the Infamous Usurping Murderers and their Families & Races, agreeable to the Just Sentence by Me pronounced against them and their Agents & Adherents, Under the special Conditions That neither Machines of Art, Air-Looms, Magnets, Magnet or other Fluids-Effluvias whether of Poisons or otherways are made Use of: Nor any Poisons or any Dastardly, Secret, or Cowardly Act be Used – . That none of the Guards, Household or Servants to them be made Use of either For if any such take part in putting them to Death I will cause them to be put to Death as Assassins on the Just Principle that although They have not any Right to Existence much less to have Guards, Households, Servants etc and although they have by their Agents been Endeavouring so many years by every Cowardly, Dastardly, poisonous, Secret, Violent, and dreadful means been Endeavouring to Murder Me and My Family; and have by such means Really Murdered My dear only Son and one of My Brothers; I will not be Assassin like their Usurping Murderous Selves nor connive at any Servant, or Person of Household, or Guard etc lifting up their hand or thought against those who have Committed themselves in Confidence to their Case etc – *But I have and hereby I do Omni Imperiously and Most Absolutely Charge and Command All Persons whomsoever Acting as Guard Household or Servants etc to any of all the said Usurping Murderers – their Families or Races by Me Pronounced against or Condemned so to declare. Respectfully and Modestly to them etc That They are Usurpers That the Territories, Sovereignty, Dominion, Power, Authority, Property etc. by them possessed or held by others for or under them etc hath belonged Originally and Antiently to My Ancestors & Family Relatives and wholly since My Birth to Me Sole and Justly; And that I have Pronounced Sentence of Death Justly against them and Commanded the Execution of such Sentence upon them; having offered Rewards for such Executing them but generously prohibited their Guards, Households & Servants etc from being made use or or taking part therein, But to disband and Return to their Own Homes and not to Serve them any Longer Under Pain of being Adjudged their Adherents & Supporters and being put to Death for the same –* And I do so further Charge and Command all such Guards, Households, Servants etc to disband themselves and Return from the Service of the said condemned; on Pain of being themselves punished with Death for the Neglect or Refusal hereof.

All Such so Refusing or Neglecting to disband themselves & Retire shall be put to Death as Supporting and Adhering to the Usurping Murderers, their Families, Races, etc And whoever Executes Death upon such as being of any of the Condemned Persons Guards, Households, or their Servants and Refusing so to disband & Retire but Persisting in their Adherence to & Support of such Usurping Murderers their Families & Races &c Shall have and Receive the Sum of One Hundred Pounds Sterling British Money or the Value thereof in other Monies paid within Three Months after My Absolute Possession of that Part of My Omni-ArchEmpire of which such so Executed were Supporting in Adhering to the Usurpation of, &c – The Awards for Executing any others so Adhering to or Supporting any of the Said Usurpers, Their Families, Races &c and of all who take possession or even Claim Possession thereof (Myself Solely Excepted) Is and shall be Twenty Pounds Sterling or the Value of other Monies to be paid for the Executing each, within Six Months at farthest after My Absolute Possession of that part of My Omni ArchEmpire in which they rendered themselves Culpable – Providing always *as a Primary Condition to all the others That every Person so Executing such Sentences has previously and publickly made his Declaration of Allegiance & Duty to Me by so Declaring That I was Born Their Absolute Sovereign, Absolute Proprietor, &c; and* that they always Persevere in such declaration And to their Utmost Assist and protect all others having so alike declared, & so alike Persevering, &c – That if any of the Usurping & Condemned are destroyed by any of the Prohibited or dastardly means, Such Part of the Awards as would have been for the Putting such so Contrary to My Commands destroyed, shall lapse from the amount one Share for each according to the Number to be Executed; And shall be distributed among the poor or withheld and not possibly be obtained by those who Receive the Remainder for Executing the others – because I will not countenance any Act which shall not be in My Estimation fair & Honourable according to My Commands – nor any Working of

Secret Assassins – But for the Executing the said Usurper fairly as by Me Commanded or Permitted of all which fair Modes I shall Prefer the Hanging them by the Neck till Dead and afterwards Publickly burning them or Severing their heads from their Dead Bodies to assure that they are Dead to be proved. The Executors shall Receive the Rewards hereafter against each Class specified, in those for each to be Executed; within Thirty days after My Absolute Possession of the said part of my OmniEmpire Territories &c

Viz: Denmark Norway &c – – Three Hundred Thousand Pounds Sterling

    Sweden &c – – – – – – – Six Hundred Thousand Pounds Sterling

    All the Russias – – – – – – – – – – One Million Pounds Sterling

    China – – – – – – – – – – – – – – One Million Pounds Sterling

All between China and Persia One Years amount of their Civil List for each –

    Persia – – – – – – – – – – – – – – One Million Pounds Sterling

    Turkey – – – – – – – – – – – – – – One Million Pounds Sterling

Africas one Years Amount of their Civil List for each; but if the Civil List of Morocco does not amount to

    Three Hundred thousand pounds Sterling: Algiers to Two Hundred Thousand Pounds Sterling; and Tunis & Tripoli to One hundred thousand pounds Sterling each; Such shall be the Sums –

Spain – – – – – – – – – – – – – – – – – – One Million Pounds Sterling

Portugal – – – – – – – – – – Three hundred thousand pounds Sterling

France – Comprizing all those who have been Actually possessed of the Sovereign & Administrative Power or pretending Right thereto Since the Eighth day of March which was in the Year One thousand Seven hundred and Sixty Six including the Soi disant Legislative & National Assemblies, Conventions, Councils, Directory, Consulate, Chief Departments of Administration and Ambassadors; Reasoning to Myself to determine respecting those who did Publicly Renounce and all Secondary & Subordinates; The Reward is Two million and a half Pounds Sterling or Sixty Millions of Livres Tournois – Supposing the Number was but Sixty it would be one Million Livres Tournois for Executing each OR if the Number was so Great as One Million (which would be less than they have destroyed!) It would be but Sixty Livres each, so that any one will befinding the Number be able to Judge what the share for each Condemneds Execution is: But this is to be Noticed That though it appears Certain that each Share in France and many other Parts will be some Hundred Pounds Sterling for Each Condemned being Executed; being somewhere between Six and Twenty thousand Livres each

Share; I have provided, That wherever the Number of Usurping Condemned is so great as that the Reward will not apportion One Hundred & Fifty Pounds Sterling for the Death of each; It shall be made up and so paid at least One hundred and Fifty Pounds Sterling or Three thousand & Six hundred Livres Tournois for the Death of each – So that If one Person Execute Ten Persons He will receive the number of Shares; And if Ten or Twenty Execute but one of the Condemned, they will have but one Share among them all.

Switzerland – those persisting in the Usurpation or pretending Right to the Exercise of Sovereignty Dominion, Power, Authority or absolute Property, or other than Subject to Me; Three hundred thousand pounds Sterling

Austria, Bohemia Hungary, & Venice, Tyrol, and so on & Sovereignty of Germany One Million of pounds Sterling

Naples & Sicily	———————	Five hundred thousand Pounds Sterling
Tuscany &c	——————————	One Hundred Thousand Pounds Sterling
Popedom	——————————	One Hundred Thousand Pounds Sterling
Sardinia &c	—————————	One Hundred Thousand Pounds Sterling
Genoa	—————————	One Hundred Thousand Pounds Sterling

Germany – One Years Civil List Amount of each Separate State for the Execution of the Usurpers thereof, their Family & Race. But for Wisternberg It is a Sum of Three hundred Thousand Pounds Sterling; For Bavaria Three Hundred Thousand Pounds Sterling: For Saxony Three hundred Thousand Pounds Sterling: And for Hanover & Bavaria separate from England Three hundred thousand Pounds Sterling – or their one Years Civil List amount at the option of the Executors Hope Cassell also Three hundred thousand pounds

Holland as for Switzerland Three hundred thousand Pounds Sterling Prussia & Brandsburg, &c Six hundred Thousand pounds Sterling Poland is Comprized in Russia & Austria, and Prussia America the Soi disant State – Five hundred Thousand Pounds Sterling British East India Company Chief in India and Soi disant Directors in England Five hundred thousand Pounds Sterling including the Commander in Chief in India & the Colonels of their Regiments in England.

British Empire; Including as follows – The Infamous Usurping Murderer George Guelph and His Family and Race –

And all those calling themselves Parliament Lords & Commons of Great Britain, Ireland &c on or since the Eight day of July

which come in the Year One Thousand Seven hundred and
Ninety Eight – And all which upon of the Soi disant Privy
Council, Cabinet, or Embassies at the said Period or have been
since then And all those Soi disant Magistrates either of Union
Hall in the Borough or of Sow Street Westminster at the End of
the Year One thousand Seven Hundred & Ninety Six, or Since
then, with all those who were calling themselves either Lord
Mayor, Aldermen, Common Council, Governors, doctor,
Apothecary, Steward, Clark, Surgeon &c of Bethlehem Hospital
on the Twenty Eight day of January which was in the Year One
thousand Seven hundred and Ninety Seven Including those
calling themselves Secretaries of State and Police Officers of
Westminster & London on the said day or Since – Including
those of the Porter Keeper at Bethlehem Hospital whom I have
Condemned for Ill treating Me, Insulting me, & Including also
all those Acting as Judges of Soi disant Law of Equity Courts
Since the said Day Including also all those Concerned in Im-
prisoning or [interfering?] with me or either of My Family
and those Exercising Power or Authority in the calling itself
College of Arms who have Witheld the [Pedigree?] of My
Family from Me & all those Concerned in Mutilating it or
who have been Suborned [?] by the Usurpers or their Agents
&c – Including also the Directors of the Bank of England, the
Stock Brokers and Loan Contractors, the Commander in Chief
of the [so] called [?] London Volunteer &c those Sycophants of
Courtiers who in defiance of My prohibiting any to go to Court
Upholding the Usurping Guelphe &c after the Thirtieth day
of January which was in the Year One thousand and Eight
hundred; have since their being dissipating My Properties,
Insulting my Right, and Publickly Courting the said Usurping
Murderous Guelphe etc and which Comprizes their Household,
& Guards refusing to Retire disband etc but for the Execution of
which Guards so Persisting in Supporting the said Usurper The
Hundred Pounds Sterling for the Death of each is more Viz
Extra The only Condition left them being so fairly to make the
declaration & Retire from their Service Ever in which Case
though they are at Liberty to take part in Extirpating the Infamous Usurping Assassins calling themselves Lords & Commons of Parliament who have so Plotted at the Murder of My
only Son and one of My Brothers and the Uncommon Efforts to
Murder Me; and though such [so] called Guards are Capable
of Receiving the Rewards for Executing such Soi disant

Introduction by Roy Porter

4 Oct 1809 Produced by ye apothecary Mr. Haslam to the House Committee   John Poynder Cl[er]k

Parliamentaries, They were totally prohibited from any Interference for or against the Infamous Guelphe & Race &c render the penalties of Death itself as mentioned – The Private Individuals who by their besetting & Ill treating Me have Encouraged the Usurpers in their dreadful Murdering Audacities against Myself & Family are also included in the Sentences to be Executed for which purpose I shall Eventually Cause them to be brought forward: But there is the Extra for Executing each.

Unfortunate for Me as it is to have to put to Death any one whomsoever; and especially such a Number; Yet it is Certain that great as this 'Number' appears, It is not half so many Persons as are literally Murdered in one Year in the Island of Great Britain only from the Effect of Machine of Art, Air Looms, Magnet, Poisons, Fluid & Effluvia etc Assortments &c in the System of Eventworking to Support there any Condemned in their Usurpation against Me – And as We all Know that every Mortal would die sometime in Course, I Notify to all my good Subjects That whenever any of the Condemned pretend That such as are Murdered by such Eventworking Infamies would die in their Turn as well as others; & That they should not Waste many Words in replying, but merely say And so would You die sometime or other if you were not now Executed – As You would live longer if Death was not Executed as a Punishment upon you, So they would have lived longer if Your Agents Assailments had not produced to them Death more early.

As for the Workers themselves especially those Gangs who have been Concerned in their Attacks on Myself and My Family; It is with me a Great Object to have them delivered up to Me alive and in their Perfect Senses, And to have their Apparatus unbroken [very?] Whole and in the State they Used it, with their Modes &c Publickly Exhibited – There is 13 or 14 in the Gang Assassinating Me, and they say Five or Six others who took part in Murdering My only Son: Several others Concerned in Murdering My Brother William and distinct Parties, who murdered My Mother & only Sister during my Infancy & Youth & Endeavoured to Murder my Father & Myself these and Four or Five Women who Endeavoured to Murder Her Omni Arch Majesty at these distant times – In order to prevent their further Atrocities & to have them delivered up to Me in their Senses Untouched, and their Machinery, Air Looms, Magnets, & whole that all My Subjects may have the Sight of them and know such weapons of Murder wherever they may be, I have determined a Separate Reward for these Purposes and so liberally as whether Ten, Twenty, Thirty, Forty, or Fifty thousand

Pounds Sterling shall be tolerable Fortune among those who Effect the apprehending & so deliver them in their Senses, and preventing their atrocities in the meanwhile.

The dreadful gang of 13 or 14 Monster Men & Women who are so making their Efforts on Me; dare every one, and boast that they have what they call Beat out of the Field Viz fairly frightened those who have approached them with a view of molesting them or even Observing them Preparatory to dragging them forth: For so dreadful are they that they would Stab mortally Virtue itself and Abash it – when any Person appears not to approve their ways much more goes near them as they say some have, they Menace them to Accuse them or their Families Wives, Daughters, Sisters, Brothers, Fathers, Sons, Selves or Relations with Murder or Concerned therein or Sodomy or Whoredom or any dreadful such like; and they say they will Revenge themselves in such manner on whoever takes part against them if they are prevented attacking them with their Machines, Air Looms, Magnets, Poisonous Effluvias &c And that if all wont believe them some will for such things uttered once are sure to find Partizans and never can be Unsaid again – Now I am of opinion that I ought to Punish instead of Pitying whoever is afraid of them or their Assassin Utterance either; for it is by such means they have arrived at that pitch of very Uncommon depravity which they have attained – Verily their common discourse much more their Furious Malice is of such Unparalelled Obscene, Filthy, dreadful Expressions & nature, as makes human Nature Shudder: But the only Cure for such Evil is to drag them forth to Public View – As the Vampiring Consequentials calling themselves the better sort but who prove to be the worst sort, are so afraid of them; the Road is open for any good Resolute fellow not Comprized in the Sentence to make His Fortune & several others also. Thus – Any such one taking about a Score good hardy Carmen, Dragmen or Countrymen; and Suddenly presenting himself and Companions at their Cavern of Rendezvous might surely be Sufficient to Outscramble such desperadoes and bring them forth – They themselves have very often declared to me, that they are in a Cellar behind the houses forming the otherside of the Street called – – – – – London Wall opposite the Middle part of Bedlam – and very often indeed Several of them have pretended that they are in an Old Subterranean place which was a pass out of the City underground when the Walls of London were existing, and that when Bedlam was Built, it was so Contrived that such Subterrane should Serve for the Workers Rendezvous and that their Apparatus is therein – that it extends under some Parts of the Building – there being an Entrance to it from some little distance through a Cellar – Sometimes others have said that they were in Upper Rooms of a house not far distant, and that their Apparatus had Conductors to every part of Bedlam and the

Neighbourhood even as far as to the Excise Office – Some of them Some-time ago also Averred that some of the calling themselves Governors of Bedlam Knew where they were well enough: but they then and at this moment say None will touch them for that all Say I am a Dangerous Man. They will find Me so to all such Assassins as themselves, their Employers and those who have Connived at their Existence: Supplied them &c. – However there cannot be a doubt but the Place of Entrance to their Rendezvous may be found – And if all other Methods fail, the letting the Water into it if it is below Ground will prevent their Using their Machine so Completely as to Injure any one – In the Magazine termed Annual Register for October Ninety one, There is an Account of the River Clyde having overflowed its Banks and I believe at Glaskow filled all the lower parts of the houses &c with Water which, reaching the lower Cells of the Madhouse where all the called Raving were, they at its approach immediately became quite Calm, even those who were the most Furious, And not only Suffered the Keepers &c to remove them up into the Upper Rooms, but remained quite Composed as long as the Water or Inundation remained – The True Secret of this was that the Water having found its way into the Place of Rendezvous of the Gang Working that Madhouse as they term it, obliged them to quit their Assassins Employ till the Water had Subsided; during which the Poor oppressed Racked, Tortured and Machine driven called Lunaticks not being assailed became as much themselves as their Machine & Magnet Agitated Rarified &c Fluids & Juices would so Immediately Admit – Their Arrivals as well as what I can Perceive prove the Certainty that this dreadful Scene of Villany of Eventworking by Working the Fluids, Juices, Brain, Vitals, Muscles, Nerves &c of Persons & their Circulations etc, is Extended to that point that in many places a Groupe of Workers are Employed in the Neighbourhoods of Private Individuals called Madmen; And that there is not a Madhouse of any Kind but to Work which there is a Gang – These Gangs have a sort of Ambassadors with other Gangs to Manage their Interests in the Actuating persons to produce Events there-from for such of the Usurping Families, Individuals, Nations, parties, persons, &c as through their Secret Agents Six or Eight fold between them and the Dirty Workers pay them Cash.

ILLUSTRATIONS

OF

MADNESS:

EXHIBITING A SINGULAR CASE OF INSANITY,

AND A NO LESS

REMARKABLE DIFFERENCE

IN

MEDICAL OPINION:

DEVELOPING

THE NATURE OF ASSAILMENT,

AND THE MANNER OF

WORKING EVENTS;

WITH A

DESCRIPTION OF THE TORTURES EXPERIENCED

BY

BOMB-BURSTING, LOBSTER-CRACKING,

AND

LENGTHENING THE BRAIN.

———

EMBELLISHED WITH A CURIOUS PLATE.

———

BY JOHN HASLAM.

" Oh! Sir, there are, in this town, Mountebanks for the mind, as well
as the body."—*Foote's Devil upon Two Sticks ; Scene the last.*

London:

PRINTED BY G. HAYDEN, BRYDGES-STREET, COVENT-GARDEN:

And Sold by

RIVINGTONS, ST. PAUL'S CHURCH-YARD; ROBINSONS, PATERNOSTER-ROW;
CALLOW, CROWN-COURT, PRINCES-STREET, SOHO;
MURRAY, FLEET-STREET; AND GREENLAND, FINSBURY-SQUARE.

———

1810.

PREFACE.

THE publication of the following case is
deemed as much an act of justice, as it
may be regarded a matter of curiosity. It
may possibly effect some good, by turning
the attention of medical men to the subject
of professional etiquette, and to a consideration of those nice feelings and reciprocal
charities, which confer on the practitioners
of medicine the amiable distinction of a
fraternity.

If it should merely succeed in curbing
the fond propensity to form hasty conclu-
sions, or tend, to moderate the mischief of

b

privileged opinion, the purpose is sufficiently answered.

From the temperate exposure of facts which the Writer has adopted, it can never be supposed that his views are hostile. The Brethren are unknown to him, and probably may never condescend to notice him beyond an occasional recollection : but if, contrary to his expectation, the Reader, throughout this narrative, should suspect a sneer, the benevolence of the Writer allows him to soften and correct it by a smile.

Of the history and opinions of the Insane, much curious matter is dispersed, and might advantageously be collected from works of various descriptions : most authors (generally without design) have contributed something ; and if such scattered materials were gleaned into a volume, the " Use and Improvement of Madness in a Commonwealth" might be sooner and more clearly ascertained.

In Germany, Mr. Spiess has published four volumes of the biography of insane

persons*, which have been perused with
much interest, and deserve to be rendered
into English : and in our own country there
exists a learned monument of madness, distinguished by abrupt transitions, a generous
reconciliation of discordant circumstances,
with a felicitous remembrance of transactions
that never occurred, and which constitute
the broad features of genuine insanity. That
the reader may duly appreciate the labours
of this gentleman, an extract is submitted
to his candid consideration †.

" I conclude with offering an interpretation of a few lines from a part of the 3d
Æneid, which, according to what is said in
my former Notes, p. 140, to which Notes I

---

* Biographien der Wahnsinnigen, von Krist. Hein-
rich Spiess, Leipzig, 1795.

† *Vide* " A Supplement to Notes on the Ancient
Method of Treating the Fever of Andalusia, now called
the Yellow Fever, deduced from an Explanation of the
Hieroglyphics painted upon the Cambridge Mummy, by
Robert Deverell, Esq. M. P. May 19, 1806," page 38.
It is a subject of regret that these scarce and luminous
pages were privately printed.

again here refer, has a particular relation to
the whole of this subject :

176   Corripio è stratis corpus, tendoque supinas
       Ad cœlum cum voce manus, et munera libo
       Intemerata focis : perfecto lætus honore
       Anchisen facio certum remque ordine pando.
       Agnovit prolem ambiguam geminosque parentes
       Seque novo veterum deceptum errore locorum.
       Tum memorat—

the meaning of which I venture to unriddle
as follows : supposing (to speak as Virgil
does, in the first person) I have a patient
attacked by a contagious pestilential disease
(its contagion being implied by the litter of
straw, è stratis, in which he lies), I take up
his body from thence, without a moment's
delay (corripio), and curry it (corripio), or
tan it (tendo), from the back and spine
(as implied perhaps by the French dos,
tergum, in tendo, and by supinas) to the
poll or hollow part of the head (that hollow part being pointed to by the Greek
word κοιλον, idem quod cœlum), or, in other
words, by administering the bark externally
to those parts (the bark being implied in
the word manus, by a reference to the

Andes), as the patient lies supine, with his face turned to the skies, in a bath which comes level with his mouth (cum voce), the great heat of which bath is denoted by (focis), as its containing an infusion of purifying aromatic herbs may be by (munera intemerata), though these words, as coupled with (libo), should at the same time seem to imply the patient's drinking a quantity of hot tea (implied perhaps by te, in intemerata). After he has thus lain in the bath a full hour (perfecto honore) with the fires that heat it well lighted, or strongly burning (lætus); I produce the effect of ensuring (facio certum) the ague-fit (implied by Anchisen, near the ice, or a fit nearly allied to ice in its nature), and thus in due order acquire a key to the fever (remque ordine pando); or these last words may perhaps imply (and then in due order resort to the use of cathartics). Of the next two lines, the first seems to intimate that the patient, in consequence of such a process, shews the twofold nature of his complaint, cold and hot, ague and fever; and the second, when

coupled with the context, that the disease
is contracted by a change of climate, viz.
that of Europe for that of the West Indies.
The two last words (tum memorat) intimate that, when that point of the process is
attained, the bark (implied by a reference
to the river Mamore, on which the tree
producing it grows) is afterwards to be
taken internally, in order to a completion
of the cure."

That the author of the Andalusia and
Supplement is a formidable rival to the spe-
cimen now to be produced, cannot in fair-
ness be denied, but in the comparison some
" partial fondness" induces me to think, that
" the superiority must, with some hesitation,
be allowed to Mr. Matthews." " If the flights
of Matthews, therefore, are higher, Deverell continues longer on the wing. Matthews often surpasses expectation, and Deverell never falls below it."

It only remains to mention that these
opinions have been collected from the
patient since the termination of the legal

proceedings; and to inform the intelligent reader that, where inverted commas are used, the manuscript of Mr. Matthews has been faithfully copied; and that, for thus introducing his philosophic opinions to the notice of a discerning public, he feels " contented and grateful."

JOHN HASLAM.

Bethlem Hospital,
  Nov. 2, 1810.

ILLUSTRATIONS

OF

MADNESS.

———

JAMES TILLY MATTHEWS, whose opinions chiefly form the subject of the following pages, was admitted a patient into Bethlem Hospital, by a petition from the parish officers of Camberwell, on the 28th of January, 1797. Although his insanity was then most evident, yet his relatives did not possess the faculty of perceiving his disorder. They employed an attorney, and by a legal process he was ordered on the second of May following to be brought to the dwelling house of the late Lord Kenyon, in Lincoln's

B

Inn Fields, who, after conversing with him, was perfectly satisfied that he was a maniac, and desired him to be remanded to his former custody. On the 21st January 1798, he was placed on the incurable establishment. In this situation he continued for many years; sometimes, an automaton moved by the agency of persons, hereafter to be introduced to the notice of the reader; at others, the Emperor of the whole world, issuing proclamations to his disobedient subjects, and hurling from their thrones the usurpers of his dominions.

In the year 1809 his relatives again interfered, and confiding in their own opinion, that he was of sound mind, and possessed the proper direction of his intellects, requested that he might be discharged. They also made application to the Churchwardens and Overseers of the parish of Camberwell, who, in the first instance, had been compelled to confine him in consequence of an order from the magistrates of Bow Street. These parish officers visited the lunatic, and being competent judges of the subject, demanded his release, on the pretence that he was perfectly recovered.

To confirm their opinion of the rational state of Mr. Matthews, the relatives employed two learned and conscientious Physicians, gentlemen deeply conversant with this disease, and doubtless instructed by copious experience to detect the finer shades and more delicate hues of intellectual disorder.

After repeated and wary examinations of the lunatic's mind, narrowly scrutinizing into his most recondite opinions, and delving into the recesses of his thoughts, they pronounced him to be perfectly in his senses, and sanctified such decision by the following affidavit, and holy affirmation.

In the King's Bench.

    HENRY CLUTTERBUCK, of Bridge Street, Blackfriars, in the City of London, Doctor of Medicine, maketh oath and saith, that he hath had four * *interviews of considerable length with James Tilly Matthews; at one* * *of which Doctor Munro was present; that this deponent could not discover any thing that indicated insanity in the said James Tilly Matthews, and he verily believes him to be perfectly sane.*

    HENRY CLUTTERBUCK.

Sworn in Court, this
Twenty-seventh Day
of November, 1809.

    By the Court.

* See (*) page 7.

In the King's Bench.

GEORGE BIRKBECK, of Cateaton Street, in the City of London, Doctor of Medicine, upon his solemn affirmation saith, that he hath paid six visits professionally to James Tilly Matthews, now under confinement in Bethlem Hospital. That during these visits he has attempted by every mode of examination which he could devise, to discover the real state of the mind of the said James Tilly Matthews, and that the result of such repeated, careful, and unprejudiced examinations, has been a conviction, that the said James Tilly Matthews is not insane. That in order to corroborate or to rectify this conclusion, he applied to Dr. Munro, the Physician to the Hospital aforesaid, for information,

*whether, by his knowledge and obser-
vation of the said James Tilly Matthews, he had been put in possession
of any particular subject or subjects,
which, on being mentioned within his
hearing, did produce maniacal hallucination, and which this affirmant
might not have been enabled to discover in the course of these conferences
with Mr. Matthews? to which question
Doctor Munro replied, that he was
not acquainted with any such subject,
but that he believed him to be insane
upon all. To render this investi-
gation more satisfactory and conclu-
sive to this affirmant, it was agreed,
that on the following Saturday he
should meet the said Doctor Munro
together, to see and converse with
Mr. Matthews. This meeting took
place accordingly; Doctor Clutterbuck (who accompanied this affirmant*

professionally in four* of the visits before mentioned)* being also present. That neither in this conference, nor in a conversation with Dr. Munro immediately subsequent thereto, (Mr. Matthews having left the room in which it took place) did any thing occur to alter the opinion of this affirmant as already expressed; but, on the contrary, that opinion was strengthened by these communications. And this affirmant further saith, that the said Dr. Munro, after finding the reasons advanced by him for the purpose of establishing the insanity of Mr. Matthews unsatisfactory to this affirmant's mind, did, near the conclusion of the interview above mentioned, declare, that although he might not succeed in convincing them, (Doctor Clutterbuck and this affirmant) or any other person, that Mr. Matthews was deranged, *he had a feeling on which he could rely, that Mr. Matthews was insane, or words of the same import. And this affirmant further saith, that the most prominent circumstances adduced in proof of the insanity of Mr. Matthews, referred to parts of his protracted confinement, not including within the last six years, with the exception of his inflexible resistance to the admission of his alledged insanity, and to the customary expression of thanks for the benefits received in the hospital, together with his unabated antipathy against the physician and apothecary, to whose care he had been entrusted during his long confinement. That the circumstances stated were not, in this affirmant's judgment, sufficient proofs of insanity, and therefore it is still the opinion and belief of this affirmant, that the mind*

*of the said James Tilly Matthews is
sound.*

GEORGE BIRKBECK.

Affirmed in Court, this⎫
   Twenty-seventh Day ⎬
of November, 1809. ⎭

By the Court.

Thus armed, the relatives moved for a
Habeas Corpus, in order that the said J. T. M.
should be discharged.

It may here be proper to state that it had
been the unvarying opinion of the medical
officers of Bethlem Hospital, that Mr. Matthews had been insane from the period of
his admission to the present time. Such
opinion was not the result of casual investi-
gation; but a conclusion deduced from daily

observation during thirteen years. But a-
ware of the fallibility of human judgment,
and suspecting that copious experience
which sheds the blessings of light upon
others, might have kept them in the dark :
perhaps startled at the powerful talents,
extensive learning, and subtile penetration
which had recorded in the face of day the
sanity of a man whom they considered as
an incurable lunatic : and flinching at an
oath contradictory to such high testimony,
the medical officers prudently referred the
determination of the case to the constituted
and best authorities in the kingdom. For
this purpose they assembled a consultation
of eminent medical practitioners, who, after
a deliberate examination of the patient's
mind, made oath in the following manner :

In the King's Bench.

SIR LUCAS PEPYS, *of Upper
Brook Street, Grosvenor Square,
in the County of Middlesex, Bart.
Doctor of Medicine, Physician to His
Majesty, President of the College of
Physicians, and one of the Commis-
sioners for visiting insane patients at
private houses;*

ROBERT DARLING WILLIS, *
of Tenterden Street, Hanover Square,
Doctor of Medicine, Fellow of the
Royal College af Physicians;*

SAMUEL FOART SIMMONS, *
of Poland Street, in the County of
Middlesex, Doctor of Medicine, Physician to St. Luke's Hospital;*

RICHARD BUDD, of Craven Street, in the Strand, Doctor of Medicine, Elect and Treasurer, and one of the Fellows of the Royal College of Physicians, and also one of the Commissioners for visiting insane patients as aforesaid;

HENRY AINSLEY, of Dover Street, Piccadilly, Doctor of Medicine, Fellow of the Royal College of Physicians, and one of the Commissioners as aforesaid;

JAMES HAWORTH, of Bedford Row, in the County of Middlesex, Doctor of Medicine, Fellow of the College of Physicians, and one of the Commissioners as aforesaid;

WILLIAM LAMBE, of the King's Road, Bedford Row, Doctor of Medi-

cine, Fellow of the Royal College of Physicians, and one of the Committee as aforesaid, (being the whole of the Commissioners appointed by the Royal College of Physicians for visiting insane persons at private houses;)

RICHARD POWELL, of Essex Street, in the Strand, Doctor of Medicine, Fellow of the Royal College of Physicians, and Secretary to the said Commissioners;

Severally make oath and say, that they had, on Wednesday, the 29th day of November instant, a long examination of the patient, James Tilley Matthews, at Bethlem Hospital, and that they took considerable pains in ascertaining the state of his mind, and that it is their positive and decided opinion, as the result of such examination, that the patient is in a most deranged state of intellect, and wholly unfit to be at large.

Sworn at my Chambers, Serjeant's Inn, by

SIR LUCAS PEPYS,
ROBERT DARLING WILLIS,
SAMUEL FOART SIMMONS,
RICHARD BUDD,
HENRY AINSLEY,
JAMES HAWORTH,
WILLIAM LAMBE,
RICHARD POWELL,

the above-named Deponents, this 30th *Day of November,* 1809, *before me,*

S. Le BLANC.

This corroboration of Mr. Matthews' insanity, by the highest and most respectable testimony, gave a different complexion to the case, and also suggested some reflections.

Madness being the opposite to reason and good sense, as light is to darkness, straight to crooked, &c. it appears wonderful that two opposite opinions could be entertained on the subject : allowing each party to possess the ordinary faculties common to human beings in a sound and healthy state, yet such is really the fact : and if one party be right, the other must be wrong : because a person cannot correctly be said to be *in* his senses and *out* of his senses at the same time.

But there is considerable difficulty and some danger in applying logic to facts. Every person who takes the degree of Doctor becomes, in consequence of taking such degree, a learned man ; and it is libellous to pronounce him ignorant. It is true, a Doctor may be blind, deaf and dumb, stupid or mad, but still his Diploma shields him from the imputation of ignorance*. It has also not unfrequently occurred, that a man who has been dubbed a Doctor of Medicine at Leyden, Aberdeen, or St. Andrews, and whose Diploma sets forth his profound learning, accomplishments, and competence to practise on the lives of His Majesty's good and faithful subjects, has been found incapable of satisfying the gentlemen in Warwick Lane that he possessed the common rudiments of his profession, and has been by them accordingly rejected : so that learning in many instances appears to be local.

Presuming Drs Birkbeck and Clutterbuck to be very learned in their profession, and,

* The feeblest intellect I ever commiserated was a Doctor of Laws from the University of Glasgow.

if possible, still more learned out of it, unit-
ing many rare talents, and distinguished by
extrinsic acquisitions,

" Grammaticus, Rhetor, Geometres, Pictor, Aliptes
" Augur, Schœnobates, Medicus, Magus——"

Conceding so much, it should follow,
that if Mr. Matthews were mad, Messrs.
Birkbeck and Co. ought to have discovered
it; but the admission of such an inference
would be destructive of their veracity: for
had they found him to be a madman, it is
to be hoped they never would stiffly and
point blank have sworn him to be in his
senses. How they could fail to detect his
insanity is inexplicable, as his disorder was
evident to all who saw and conversed with
him; even his fellow-*students* * derided the
absurdity of his doctrine:—however, it
should be recollected that these gentlemen

c

* Is any *student* tearing his straw in piece-meal,
swearing and blaspheming, biting his grate, foaming at
the mouth, &c.—*Vide Tale of a Tub, page* 178, *edit.*
1704.

have much practical experience, and are competent judges of all systems of error but their own.

It appears, these Doctors generally visited him in conjunction: perhaps they might have succeeded better, if they had examined him separately; for it is within the range of possibility that the judgment may have been warped by the courtesy, or clouded by the formality of a consultation—

" As two spent swimmers,
" That do cling together, and choke their art."

It may here be allowable to state, that if Drs. Birkbeck and Co. had, in the first instance, made application to the medical officers of the hospital, and announced their object, they would have been received with the urbanity due to professional gentlemen, and furnished with every information; but they preferred a silent approach and secret inquisition.

In the ordinary language of our courts of law, the relatives took nothing by their motion; nor is it my intention to bestow a single sentence on their conduct— the practice of the two Doctors shall be left to the humane construction of the Christian reader; and to finish the paragraph, the churchwardens and overseers of the parish of Camberwell may be supposed to have acted most conscientiously; and that the convenience of being disburthened of a pauper lunatic never entered their thoughts.

I shall now proceed to develope the peculiar opinions of Mr. Matthews, and leave the reader to exercise his own judgment concerning them.

———————

Mr. M. insists that in some apartment near London Wall, there is a gang of villains profoundly skilled in Pneumatic Chemistry, who assail him by means of an Air

Loom. A description of this formidable instrument will be given hereafter; but he is persuaded that an account of it is to be found in Chambers's Dictionary, edited by Dr. Rees in 1783, under the article *Loom*, and that its figure is to be seen in one of the plates relating to Pneumatics.

It is unnecessary to tell the reader that he will fruitlessly search that work for such information.

The assailing gang consits of seven members, four of whom are men and three women. Of these persons four are commonly resident, and two have never stirred abroad since he has been the subject of their persecution. Of their general habits little is known; occasionally they appear in the streets, and by ordinary persons would be taken to be pick-pockets or private distillers. They leave home to correspond with others of their profession; hire themselves out as spies, and discover the secrets of government to the enemy, or confederate to work events of the most atrocious nature. At home they lie together in promiscuous intercourse and filthy community

The principal of this crew, is named Bill, or the King : he formerly surpassed the rest in skill, and in the dexterity with which he worked the machine : he is about 64 or 5 years of age, and in person resembles the late Dr. De Valangin, but his features are coarser; perhaps, he is a nearer likeness to the late Sir William Pultney, to whom he is made a duplicate. It was on account of something worked by this wretch, that another, by the force of *assailment**, actuated Rhynwick Williams to the commisssion of his monstrous practices. He also took Hadfield in

* This term, which frequently occurs, and is not to be found in our dictionaries, either originates with Mr. M. or is extracted from the vocabulary of the pneumatic gang.

tow, by means of magnetic impregnations, and compelled him to fire the Pistol at His Majesty in the theatre : but on this subject there is a difference of opinion, as some of the female part of the gang attribute this event to *Blue-Mantle*, of whom nothing farther is known. In working the machine Bill exerts the most unrelenting and murderous villany ; and he has never been observed to smile.

The next in order, is a being called *Jack the Schoolmaster*, who is the short-hand-writer to the gang : he styles himself the recorder ; somewhat tall, and about 60 years of age. It is not well ascertained if he wear a wig, but he generally appears in the act of shoving his wig back with his fore-finger, and frequently says, " So you shall, when you can ketch (catch) us at it." Sometimes he says, " I'm to see fair play," and makes a merriment of the business. Jack has very seldom worked the machine.

The third person is *Sir Archy*, who is about 55 years of age, wears a drab-coloured coat, and, according to the old fashion, his breeches button between the legs. Some of the gang assert that Sir Archy is a woman dressed in men's apparel; and whenever Mr. Matthews has endeavoured, by enquiry, to ascertain this fact, Sir Archy has answered in a manner so quaint and indelicate that I cannot venture to communicate his reply. He is considered as the common liar of the gang; a low-minded blackguard, always cracking obscene jokes and throwing out gibes and sarcasms. In his speech there is an affectation of a provincial accent, so that when Mr. M. asserts the truth of any fact, Sir Archy replies yho (you) are misteaken mistaken) He constantly stays in the apartment, and says he does not work the machine, but only uses a magnet. His mode of communicating with Mr. M. is principally by " *brain-*

sayings," which term will be afterwards explained.

The last of the males is termed the *Middle Man*, who is about 57 years of age, of the middle stature, with a broad chest; has a twang of the hawk countenance, not pockfretten, and much resembling the late Mr. Smeaton the engineer. He is dressed in a blue coat, with a plain waistcoat. It is said that he is a manufacturer of air-looms, and possesses the first rate skill in working this instrument. Altho' he is unrelenting in his persecution of Mr. M. he appears to consider it as sport, and sits grinning, apparently delighted that he cannot be taken unawares. After his attacks, he generally observes that Mr. M. is the talisman; then Sir Archy replies, with a sneer, " Yes, he is the talisman."

Among the females who compose this

establishment, *Augusta* may first be described. She is about 36 years of age, of the middle stature, and her countenance is distinguished by the sharpness of its features. In person she is not fleshy, nor can she be said to be a thin woman; she is not full-breasted. Ordinarily dressed, as a country tradesman's wife, in black, without powder. Augusta seldom works the machine, but frequently goes abroad to correspond with other gangs at the West end of the town. Of agreeable deportment, and at first seems very friendly and cajoling; but when she finds that she cannot influence and convince, becomes exceedingly spiteful and malignant. Her object is to influence women by her brain-sayings; and she states herself to be the chief of this department. Within the last seven years the virulence of her temper has been considerably exasperated.

Charlotte, the next in review, is about the

same age as Augusta, and also of the middle
stature, but more fleshy; has the appearance of a French woman, being a kind of
ruddy brunette. She constantly stays at
home with Sir Archy, and complains that
she is forcibly confined to this situation.
They keep her nearly naked, and poorly fed.
Mr. Matthews is led to suppose that she is
chained; for she has sometimes stated herself to be equally a prisoner with himself.
Charlotte always speaks French, but her
language and brain-sayings are conveyed in
an English idiom. Her character is that of
a steady, persevering sort of person, who is
convinced of the impropriety of her conduct, but cannot help herself. For several
years she has not worked the machine, but
is a fixed and established reporter.

A very extraordinary lady compleats this
malicious group. She does not appear to
have any Christian name, but by the gang

is termed the *Glove Woman*, as she constantly wears cotton-mittens. Sir Archy dryly insinuates that she keeps her arms thus covered because she has got the itch. She is about 48 years of age, is above the middle height, and has a sharp face. On her chin and upper lip there is a considerable quantity of fine downy hair, and she is somewhat pockfretten. Always dressed in a common fawn-coloured Norwich gown, with a plain cream-coloured camblet shawl, and wears a chip hat covered with black silk. The glove woman is remarkable for her skill in managing the machine. She frequently goes abroad. The rest of the gang, but particularly Sir Archy, are constantly bantering and plucking at her, like a number of rooks at a strange jack-daw : she has never been known to speak.

Having described the *dramatis personæ*, it is expedient to mention the different preparations which are employed in the air-loom, by these pneumatic adepts, for the purposes of assailment.

Seminal fluid, male and female — Effluvia of copper — ditto of sulphur — the vapours of vitriol and aqua fortis — ditto of nightshade and hellebore — effluvia of dogs — stinking human breath — putrid effluvia — ditto of mortification and of the plague — stench of the sesspool — gaz from the anus of the horse — human gaz — gaz of the horse's greasy heels — Egyptian snuff, (this is a dusty vapour, extremely nauseous, but its composition has not been hitherto ascertained*) — vapour and effluvia of arsenic—

---

* This disgusting odour is exclusively employed during sleep, when, by their *dream-workings*, they have placed him, as a solitary wanderer, in the marshes near the mouth of the river Nile ; not at that season when its waters bring joy and refreshment, but at its lowest ebb, when the heat is most oppressive, and the

poison of toad—otto of roses and of car-
nation.

The effects which are produced on Mr.
Matthews by the skilful manipulation of
these ingredients are according to his relation dreadful in the extreme.   He has stated
them in the technical language of the
assailing gang, and explained their operation on his intellect and person.   Whoever
peruses a work on Nosology will be pain-
fully impressed with its formidable catalogue
of human miseries; it therefore becomes
exceedingly distressing to swell the volume
with a list of calamities hitherto unheard

muddy and stagnant pools diffuse a putrid and suffocat-
ing stench ;—the eye is likewise equally disgusted with
the face of the country, which is made to assume a hate-
ful tinge, resembling the dirty and cold blue of a scor-
butic ulcer.   From this cheerless scene they suddenly
awake him, when he finds his nostrils stuffed, his mouth
furred, and himself nearly choaked by the poisonous
effects of their Egyptian snuff.

of, and for which no remedy has been yet discovered.

Fluid Locking.—A locking or constriction of the fibres of the root of the tongue, laterally, by which the readiness of speech is impeded.

Cutting soul from sense.—A spreading of the magnetic warp, chilled in its expansion, from the root of the nose, diffused under the basis of the brain, as if a veil were interposed; so that the sentiments of the heart can have no communication with the operations of the intellect.

Stone-making.—The gang pretend they can at pleasure produce a precipitation in the bladder of any person impregnated, and form a calculus. They boast of having effected this in a very complete manner for the late Duke of Portland.

Thigh-talking.—To effect this, they contrive so to direct their *voice-sayings* on the
external part of the thigh, that the person
assailed is conscious that his organ of hearing, with all its sensibility, is lodged in that
situation. The sensation is distinctly felt in
the thigh, and the subject understood in the
brain.

Kiteing.—This is a very singular and distressing mode of assailment, and much practised by the gang. As boys raise a kite in
the air, so these wretches, by means of the
air-loom and magnetic impregnations, contrive to lift into the brain some particular
idea, which floats and undulates in the intellect for hours together; and how much
soever the person assailed may wish to
direct his mind to other objects, and banish
the idea forced upon him, he finds himself
unable; as the idea which they have kited
keeps waving in his mind, and fixes his at-

tention to the exclusion of other thoughts.
He is, during the whole time, conscious that
the kited idea is extraneous, and does not
belong to the train of his own cogitations.

Sudden death-squeezing; by them termed
Lobster-cracking.—This is an external pressure of the magnetic atmosphere surround-
ing the person assailed, so as to stagnate his
circulation, impede his vital motions, and
produce instant death.

" In short, I do not know any better
way for a person to comprehend the
general nature of such lobster-cracking
operation, than by supposing himself in a
sufficiently large pair of nut-crackers or
lobster-crackers, with teeth, which should
pierce as well as press him through every
particle within and without ; he expe-
riencing the whole stress, torture, driving,
oppressing, and crush all together."

Stomach-skinning consists in rendering the stomach raw and sore, as if it had been scalded, and the internal coat stripped off.

Apoplexy-working with the nutmeg-grater consists in violently forcing the fluids into the head; and where such effort does not suddenly destroy the person, producing small pimples on the temples, which are raised, and rough like the holes in a nutmeg-grater: in a day or two they gradually die away.

Lengthening the brain.—As the cylindrical mirror lengthens the countenance of the person who views himself in such glass, so the assailants have a method by which they contrive to elongate the brain. The effect produced by this process is a distortion of any idea in the mind, whereby that which had been considered as most serious

D

becomes an object of ridicule. All thoughts
are made to assume a grotesque interpretation ; and the person assailed is surprised
that his fixed and solemn opinions should
take a form which compels him to distrust
their identity, and forces him to laugh at
the most important subjects. It can cause
good sense to appear as insanity, and convert truth into a libel ; distort the wisest
institutions of civilized society into the practices of barbarians, and strain the Bible into
a jest book.

Thought-making.—While one of these
villains is sucking at the brain of the person
assailed, to extract his existing sentiments,
another of the gang, in order to lead astray
the sucker (for deception is practised among
themselves as a part of their system ; and
there exists no honor, as amongst thieves, in
the community of these rascals) will force
into his mind a train of ideas very different

from the real subject of his thoughts, and
which is seized upon as the desired information by the person sucking; whilst he
of the gang who has forced the thought on
the person assailed, laughs in his sleeve at
the imposition he has practised.

Laugh-making consists in forcing the
magnetic fluid, rarified and subtilized, on
the vitals, [*vital touching*] so that the
muscles of the face become screwed into a
laugh or grin.

Poking, or *pushing up the quicksilver.*—
When the person assailed possesses an intellect sufficiently strong to be conscious of
his impregnation, he naturally revolts at
the atrocities practised upon him by the
workers of this infernal machine, and becomes prompted to express his indignation
at their perfidy. While in the act, as he
supposes, of venting the burst of indigna-

tion, they contrive to push a seeming thread
of fluid through his back diagonally in the
direction of his vitals.   Its operation is in-
stantaneous, and the push appears to elevate
the fluid about half an inch.   This magic
touch disarms the expression of his resent-
ment, and leaves him an impotent prey to
the malignity of their scorn and ridicule.

Bladder-filling is filling the nerves of
the neck with gaz, and by continued distension, effecting a partial dislocation of the
brain.   This frequently repeated, produces
weakness of intellect.

Tying-down; fettering the energy of the
assailed's judgment on his thoughts.

Bomb-bursting is one of the most dreadful
inflictions performed by the infernal agency
of the air-loom.   The fluid which resides in
the brain and nerves. the vapor floating in

ILLUSTRATIONS OF MADNESS.

the blood-vessels, and the gaz which occu-
pies the stomach and intestines, become
highly rarified and rendered inflammable,
occasioning a very painful distension over
the whole body. Whilst the assailed person is thus labouring, a powerful charge of
the electrical battery (which they employ
for this purpose) is let off, which produces
a terrible explosion, and lacerates the whole
system. A horrid crash is heard in the head,
and if the shock do not prove instantly
fatal, the party only recovers to express
his astonishment that he has survived the
murderous attempt.

Gaz-plucking is the extraction of magnetic fluid from a person assailed, such fluid
having been rarified and sublimed by its
continuance in the stomach and intestines.
This gaz is in great request, and considered
as the most valuable for the infernal purposes of these wretches. They contrive, in a

very dexterous manner, to extract it from the anus of the person assailed, by the suction of the air-loom. This process is performed in a very gradual way, bubble by bubble.

The explanation of the forementioned terms will enable the reader sufficiently to understand others which belong to the science of assailment, as *foot-curving*, *lethargy-making*, *spark-exploding*, *knee-nailing*, *burning out*, *eye-screwing*, *sight-stopping*, *roof-stringing*, *vital-tearing*, *fibre-ripping*, &c. &c. &c.

The correspondence between Mr. M. and the members of this gang is kept up to a considerable extent by *brain-sayings*, which may be defined a sympathetic communication of thought, in consequence of both parties being impregnated with the magnetic fluid, which must be rarified by frequent changing, and rendered more powerful by the action of the electrical machine. It is not hearing; but appears to be a silent conveyance of intelligence to the intellectual atmosphere of the brain, as subtilely as electricity to a delicate electrometer: but the person assailed (if he be sufficiently strong in intellect) is conscious that the perception is not in the regular succession of his own thoughts. The first hint Mr. M. received of the possibility of such sympathetic communication was in France, before the period of his confinement. He there, in one of the prisons, became acquainted with a Mr. Chavanay, whose father had been cook to Lord Lonsdale. One day, when they were sitting together, Mr. Chavanay said, "Mr. Matthews, are you acquainted with the art of talking with your brains?" Mr. M. replied in the negative. Mr. C. said, "It is effected by means of the magnet."

They likewise impart their thoughts to him by *voice-sayings*. This is an immediate conveyance of articulate sound to the auditory nerves, without producing the ordinary vibrations of air; so that the communication is intelligibly lodged in the cavity of the ear, whilst the bystander is not sensible of any impression.

Even during sleep they contrive to annoy him with their *dream-workings*, which consist in the power they exert of forcing their phantoms and grotesque images on his languid intellect. These assassins hold in their possession puppets of uncouth shape, and of various descriptions; by looking steadily at which they can throw the form into his brain, and thus render the perception more vivid to the dreamer; and the crafty solicitude with which they glean his waking opinions on the mysteries which, during the night, have danced in his imagination, is both wonderful and distressing.

On some occasions Mr. M. has been able to discern them ; but whenever he has been watching their manœuvres, and endeavouring to ascertain their persons minutely, they have appeared to *step back*, and eluded his search, so that a transient glimpse could only be obtained.

" Diffugient comites, et nocte tegentur opaca."

But the gang relate that they do not actually step back ; but, at the moment when they are observed, that they grasp a metal which has the power of weakening the sympathy between them and the person assailed, and of benumbing his perception. This metal appears to be formed like a distaff or truncheon, and two such are fixed on the top of the machine. At other times, they have pretended that each member of the gang is furnished with a separate metal.

The annexed figure of the air-loom, sketched by Mr. Matthews, together with *his* explanations, will afford the necessary information concerning this curious and wonderful machine.

REFERENCES.

" *a a.* The top of the apparatus, called by the assassins air-loom machine, pneumatic machine, &c. being as a large table.

" *b b.* The metals which the workers grasp to deaden the sympathy.

" *c.* The place where the pneumaticians sit to work the loom.

" *d.* Something like piano-forte keys, which open the tube valves within the air-

loom, to spread or feed the warp of magnetic fluid.

" *e e.* Levers, by the management of which
the assailed is wrenched, stagnated, and the
sudden-death efforts made upon him, &c.
The levers are placed at those points of
elevation, *viz.* the one nearly down, at
which I begin to let go my breath, taking
care to make it a regular, not in any way a
hurried breathing. The other, the highest,
is where it begins to strain the warp, and
by which time it becomes necessary to have
taken full breath, to hold till the lever was
so far down again. This invariably is the
vital-straining. But in that dreadful operation by them termed lobster-cracking, I always found it necessary to open my mouth
somewhat sooner than I began to take in
breath ; I found great relief by so doing,
and always imagined, that as soon as the
lever was at the lowest, (by which time I

had nearly let go my breath) the elasticity of the fluid about me made it recoil from the forcible suction of the loom, much in the manner as a wave recoils or shrinks back after it has been forced forward on the sands in the ebbing or flowing of the tide : and then remains solely upon its own gravity, till the general flux or stress again forces it forward in form of a wave. Such appears to me the action of the fluid, which, from the time the lever being fully down, loses all suction-force upon it. I always thought that by so opening my mouth, which many strangers, and those familiar or about me, called sometimes singularity, at others affectation and pretext, and at others asthmatic, &c. instantly let in such momentarily emancipated fluid about me, and enabled me sooner, easier, and with more certainty, to fill my lungs without straining them, and this at every breathing.

" *f.* Things, apparently pedals, worked by the feet of the pneumaticians.

" *g.* Seemingly drawers, forming part of the apparatus as eudiometer, &c. &c.

" *h.* The cluster of upright open tubes or cylinders, and by the assassins termed their *musical glasses,* which I have so often mentioned, and perceived when they were endeavouring to burst my person, by exploding the interior of the cavity of the trunk. I now find an exact likeness in the Cyclopedia, which, being in electricity, is termed a battery.

" *i.* The apparatus mentioned as standing upon the air-loom, which the assassins were ever so watchful and active, by deadening the sympathy, to prevent my holding sight of; so that I could never ascertain what the bulky upper parts were, although the lower parts have appeared as distinct as the strength of the drawing shews. But I never had longer than the slow-glimpse-sight.

" *k l m.* The bulky upper parts, which, though always indistinct, appeared once or twice to be hid by an horizontal broad projection, and which has often made me query whether they rose through an aperture of the cellar ceiling into the room above, which the assassins' brain-sayings have frequently seemed to acknowledge.

" *n.* The windmill kind of sails I have so often mentioned, only seen by the glimpse of sympathy ; and to prevent my judging of which, the assassins would dash with full strong sympathy or brain-saying, ' a whirligig,' used by children for amusement. But such windmill ever appeared as standing on the table.

" *o.* The barrels, which I perceived so distinctly after such long watching, to catch the sight of the famous goose-neck-retorts, which, by the assassins, are asserted to be about their loom, for supplying it with the distilled gazes, as well poisoned as magnetic, but which did not expose the goose-necks, which are here given, to shew the kind the assassins have, during ten years, some thousand times asserted they had : for while I was dwelling upon retorts themselves, which I had expected to find of metal, as stills, but which appeared distinctly hooped barrels standing on end on the floor, they cut the sympathy, and have ever since at all my attempts dashed or splashed the inward nerves of vision to bully and baffle me out of it.

" *p q r.* That part of the brass apparatus, so often seen distinctly of bright brass, standing on a one step-high boarded floor, having a bright iron railing around it, the part not here shewn was never distinct.

" s s. The warp of magnetic-fluid, reaching between the person impregnated with such fluid, and the air-loom magnets to which it is prepared ; which being a multiplicity of fine wires of fluid, forms the sympathy, streams of attraction, repulsion, &c. as putting the different poles of the common magnet to objects operates ; and by which sympathetic warp the assailed object is affected at pleasure : as by open-ing a vitriolic gaz valve he becomes tortured by the fluid within him ; becoming agitated with the corrosion through all his frame, and so on in all their various modes of attacking the human body and mind, whether to actuate or render inactive ; to make ideas or to steal others ; to bewilder or to deceive ; thence to the driving with

rage to acts of desperation, or to the drop-
ping dead with stagnation, &c. &c. &c.
Though so distinct to me by sympathy I
have never caught the inward vision thereof,
not even by glimpse; but the assassins
pretend, when heated, that it becomes
luminous and visible to them for some yards
from the loom, as a weakish rainbow, and
shews the colours according to the nature
of the gazes from which it is formed, or
wherewith the object is impregnated: as
green for the copper-streams or threads, red
for the iron, white for the spermatic animal-
seminal, &c.

" *t.* Shews the situation of the repeaters,
or active worriers, when such were employed during the active exertions so long
made to worry me down.

" *u.* One of the assassins called by the

E

rest Jack the Schoolmaster, who calls his exertions to prevent my writing or speaking correctly, *dictating*, he ever intruding his own style and endeavouring to force it upon me. He pretends to be the short-hand-writer, to register or record every thing which passes. He appears to have a seat with a desk some steps above the floor.

" V. The female of the gang called by the others Charlotte: she has always spoken French, even by her brain-sayings; but I yet doubt whether she be a French woman, though so much of that description of person, for frequently it is English-French: though this may be from *their* vocabulary being English and French combined.

" W. The one I call the common liar of the gang, by them termed Sir Archy, who often speaks in obscene language. There has never been any fire in the cellar where the machinery is placed.

" X. Suppose the assailed person at the greater distance of several hundred feet, the warp must be so much longer directly towards him, but the farther he goes from the pneumatic machine, the weaker becomes its hold of him, till I should think at one thousand feet he would be out of danger. I incline to think that at such distance or little more, the warp would break, and that the part nearest his person would withdraw into him, and that next the loom would shrink into whatever there held it.

" Y. The middle man working the air-loom, and in the act of Lobster-cracking the person represented by the figure X.

" The assassins say they are not five hundred feet from me ; but from the uncommon

force of all their operations, I think they
are much nearer."

They have likewise related that many
other gangs are stationed in different parts
of the metropolis who work such instrument for the most detrimental purposes.
Near every public office an air-loom is concealed, and if the police were sufficiently
vigilant, they might detect a set of wretches
at work near the Houses of Parliament,
Admiralty, Treasury, &c. and there is a
gang established near St. Luke's Hospital.
The force of assailment is in proportion
to the proximity of the machine; and it
appears that the interposition of walls
causes but a trifling difference : perhaps at
the distance of 1000 feet a person might be
considered out of the range of its influence.
Independently of the operation of this complex and powerful machine termed an Air-
loom, which requires the person assailed to

be previously saturated with magnetic fluid, a number of emissaries, who are termed *novices*, are sent about in different directions to prepare those who may hereafter be employed in the craft and mystery of event-working. This is termed *Hand-impregnation*, and is effected in the following manner: an inferior member of the gang, (generally a novice,) is employed in this business. He is furnished with a bottle containing the magnetic fluid which issues from a valve on pressure. If the object to be assailed be sitting in a coffee-house, the pneumatic practitioner hovers about him, perhaps enters into conversation, and during such discourse, by opening the valve, sets at liberty the volatile magnetic fluid which is respired by the person intended to be assailed. So great is the attraction between the human body and this fluid, that the party becomes certainly impregnated, and is equally bound by the spell as the lady was fixed to the chair of Comus, or the harmless fly is enveloped in the shroud of the spider.

In order to ascertain whether a person be impregnated, let him, fasting, imitate the act of swallowing, and if he should perceive a grating noise in his ears, somewhat resembling the compression of a new wicker-basket he is certainly attained.

In consequence of the numerous gangs established in this metropolis, all the persons holding high situations in the government are held impregnated. An expert of the gang, who is magnetically prepared, contrives to place himself near the person of a minister of state also impregnated, and is thus enabled to force any particular thought into his mind and obtain his reflections on the thought so forced.—Thus, for instance, when a Secretary at War is at church, in the theatre, or sitting in his office and thinking on indifferent subjects; the expert magnetist

would suddenly throw into his mind the
subject of exchange of prisoners. The
Secretary would, perhaps, wonder how he
became possessed of such a subject, as it
was by no means connected with his
thoughts; he would however turn the topic
in his mind and conclude that such particular principle ought to form the basis of
the negociation. The expert magnetist,
having, by watching and sucking, obtained
his opinion, would immediately inform the
French Minister of the sentiments of the
English Secretary, and by such means become enabled to baffle him in the exchange.

The same process would take place with the
other ministers of state, and their opinions
would be communicated to the enemy on
the subjects of peace, commercial intercourse,
or the fitting out of armaments. Let the
plan be ever so well devised, the magnetists
would be certain to paralize and bewilder

the person chosen to command the expedi-
tion.   This they effected in a very complete
manner at Buenos Ayres, and still more recently in the Island of Walcheren.

Notwithstanding the dreadful sufferings
which Mr. Matthews experiences from being
assailed, he appears to derive some consolation
from the sympathy which prevails between
himself and the workers of the machine.—
Perilous as his present situation may be, it
would be rendered still more alarming if he
could not watch their proceedings, and thus
be prepared to avert the force of their engine.
This reciprocal impregnation and conti-
nuity of warp enables him to perceive *their*
motions and attain *their* thoughts. Such
seems to be the law of this sympathy, that
mutual intelligence is the result ; nor can the
assailants, with all their skill and dexterity,
deprive him of this corresponding perception.
In proportion as their scientific advancement

has instructed them in new and ingenious arts of tormenting, the progression of his experience has taught him to diminish the force of their attacks.

These assassins are so superlatively skillful in every thing which relates to pneumatic chemistry, physiology, nervous influence, sympathy, human mind, and the higher metaphysic, that whenever their persons shall be discovered, and their machine exhibited, the wisest professors will be astonished at their progress, and feel ashamed at their own ignorance. The gang proudly boast of their contempt for the immature science of the present æra.

Under all these persecutions and formidable assailments, it is the triumph of Mr. M. that he has been enabled to sustain himself; and this resistance has depended on the strength of his intellect and unremitting

vigilance. Whenever he has perceived
them about to make the wrench by suction,
he has recoiled as one expecting to receive
a blow shrinks back in order to avoid it.
Without such ability and precaution he must
long since have become the victim of
bomb-bursting, lobster-cracking, or apoplexy-working with the nutmeg-grater.

Having described the machinery and
actors in this " insubstantial pageant" it now
only remains to afford some idea of the nature of *Event-working*, a science formerly
supposed to depend on certain positions of
the planetary system, and regulated by
heads of houses in the university of the
stars. Although much attention and some
valuable time have been lost in becoming
acquainted with this novel philosophy, yet
after repeated trials and painful efforts, the
writer has been unable adequately to explain
the manner of working an event, particularly

as the event is commemorated before it
occurs. From these embarrassments he has
been kindly relieved by Mr. Matthews, who
has written down his ideas on the subject,
and from whose manuscript the following
pages are exhibited to the reader.

" The assassins opened themselves by their
voices to me about Michaelmas 1798, and
for several years called their infamies,
working feats of arms, but seldom using the
term *Event-working :* though after four or
five years, when I, by perseverance, had
beat them out of their insolence of assumption, (for they assumed the right of interfering with every body having heraldic
bearings particularly, and for this part of
their villanies called themselves the *efficient
persons* to all those having titles to colleges
of arms,) and *by* such titles also they used
the term event-working for their actions.

" It is not an easy matter to define fully
any regular instance of such, their called
event-working, because they in every thing
introduced the names of some, or other per-
sonages, as concerned therewith, but who
certainly, were not only ignorant of their
very existence, but more or less victims to
their abominations.

" However, to shew what the nature of
such event-working is, namely, how infamous human beings, making a profession of
pneumatic chemistry, and pneumatic mag-
netism, hire themselves as spies; and by
impregnating persons, singled out by them as
objects for interfering with, obtaining their
secrets, actuating them in various ways, in
thought, word and deed, as well as they can,
to model their conduct, ideas or measures to
favour the ends of assassin spies or event-
workers, or their employers, &c. in bringing
about which ends they sometimes are years

and many years, varying from mode to mode from stratagem to stratagem, and sometimes partially fail at last, according to the difficulty of getting near the object to operate upon, the strength of such person's nerves, brain, and personal affections, as well as nature of soul, &c. &c. The following, divested of their offensive introductions may suffice, being a few instances out of numberless events.

" While I was detained in Paris by the then existing French Government, during the years 1793-4-5, and beginning of 1796, I had even in the early part thereof, suffi- cient information, to be certain that a regular plan existed, and was furthering by persons in France, connected with persons in Eng- land, as well for surrendering to the French every secret of the British Government, as for the republicanizing Great Britain and Ireland, and particularly for disorganizing the British navy ; to create such a confusion therein, as to admit the French armaments to move without danger.

" My sentiments having been resolutely hostile to every such plan, idea, and person assisting therein, proved, (as the assassins have ever avowed) the real cause of my having had Gens d'armes placed with me to prevent my return, and their having by such magnetic means of workers in Paris ascertained, that my said sentiments were so determined for the counteracting such plans, as well as others more dreadful in their nature, that I should persevere even to the loss of my life in my efforts to expose them. They have ever avowed also; that my having immediately on my return set about exposing the quoted infamies, occasioned a magnetic spy to be appointed from each gang of event-workers in London, specially to watch and circumvent me : for that the chiefs of such gangs were the real persons who were

clokcd under certain names and titles used
in the information given me, and which I
have for years found such vile spy-traitor-
assassins called by among their fraternity.

"That the persons mentioned by me in my
letters, narratives, &c. to each of the 1796
administration, and to the then Speaker of the
House of Commons as spies, whom I could
not discover, but found, as it were, before
me, behind me, and on every side of me,
every where, and in every thing (as was my
expression) were magnetic spy-workers
coming from Paris, at the time I was trudg-
ing it from thence, and having the charge
of circumventing me; and such were so
appointed by each of the London gangs,
event-working assassins: who having found
my senses proof against their fluid and hand-
working, as it is termed, were employed to
actuate the proper persons to pretend I was
insane, for the purpose of plunging me into

a madhouse, to invalidate all I said, and for the purpose of confining me within the measure of the Bedlam-attaining-airloom-warp, making sure that by means thereof, and the poisonous effluvia they used, they would by such means keep me fully impregnated, and which impregnation could be renewable and aggravated at their pleasure, so as to overpower my reason and speech, and destroy me in their own way, while all should suppose it was insanity which produced my death.

That not only such appointed spies, but the whole phalanx of event-workers, all the gangs rose up in arms against me; because all depended during that year (1796) on their disorganizing the British navy, which they had undertaken to effect, and had their experts at work to bring about; while my incessant and loud clamours, almost daily writing to, or calling at the houses of one or

other of all the ministers in their turn, con-
juring them to exert themselves to prevent
wretches from disorganizing the British
navy; this obliged such experts and gangs
also, to have recourse to such caution till
they could get rid of me; that in truth, they
could not make any way therein while I
was at large : and to this solely was owing
their not having been able to fulfil their
engagements with the French, to have the
British fleet in confusion by the time stipulated; and which inability from such fear,
more than the storm, forced General Hoche,
whose armament was called the Avant-Garde
of the intended French invasion to return as
he came. And they have ever pretended
that Hoche, having been exasperated against
the workers, spoke bitterly of them, and
was by one of their experts *put out:* (viz.
destroyed by poisonous magnetic fluid, which
kills by possessing itself of the hollows of

the nerves, and does not affect the stomach, vitals, &c. as poysons in substance,) in order to prevent him from publishing the existence of the profession.

" That finding it much easier to actuate all the ministers, magistrates, &c. to the folly of pretending me mad, than to make me desist from exerting myself to expose the plots and plans of such assassins, they adopted this course, and at last contrived my being forced into Bedlam, where they have ever sworn, they will by hook or by crook hold me ; and some thousand times during the last twelve years, sworn I should never get out of their clutches alive, unless I forgave them ; but they know all compromise with them is impossible.

" That having me safely immured, the experts went to work again boldly, and then, in less than three months blew up that flame in the British navy, which threw the three great fleets into open mutiny, about Easter 1797 : that this proving to the then ministry their danger, from their having mocked, and (by their tools, which as well as the ministers themselves, were tools in the hands of event-working assassins) imprisoned me; they then became so alarmed on the second mutiny of the Nore fleet, under Parker, a man actuated by magnet-working experts, that they opened the Treasury doors, and instead of attending to me, cost the nation near one hundred thousand pounds in secret service money, to quell the mutiny at the Nore, and prevent its again bursting out at Portsmouth, Plymouth, &c. and that to avoid the expenditure being noticed, as such, means were contrived to work it into the accounts, as for other purposes at earlier periods.

" It has ever been their custom to actuate

every one to insult or ill-treat me: they
could give their time to actuate, and then
to swear to avenge it, and make a merit of
event-working, to bring disgrace or injury
upon such persons: never indeed, to benefit
me; but as pursuing their systems of villany, calling me their *Property* and *Talisman,* bringing persons under what they call
their *Fluid-balances* against me; perse-
cuting and making murderous efforts upon
me: using the name or expression, or the
presence of particular persons as their authority, and then pretending, because I with-
stood them, that they had a right against
such persons, or whom they called such
persons duplicates to.

" Hence they ever asserted that Mr. Pitt
was not half able to withstand magnetic
fluid in its operative effect, but became
actuated like a mere puppet by the expert-
magnetists employed in such villanies:

that every one of his colleagues and suc-
cessors to the present moment, have proved
equally actuable, though some more, some
less, Mr. Grey having proved the strongest,
though not full proof : and pretending in
their efforts to cajole me, that my having,
(though not acquainted with him, and notwithstanding his refusing to attend to *me* in
1796,) entertained a sort of friendly opinion
for him, was the sole means of preserving his
life when first Lord of the Admiralty. They
say, that having read in my jumbled narratives
the facts of traitor efforts to disorganize the
navy, and even after the meeting, not only
left me to linger here under their incessant
murdering efforts, but accepted the office of
first Lord of the Admiralty ; the die was
cast against him in their system of event-
working, and he was to be *put out*, a term
they use for their murdering any one. In
truth, they did frequently say to me, when
he took upon him the office, ‘ *We have*

event-worked that ; he is to be killed there :'
and I mentioned it to several : but as all des-
pised me and said it was insanity, I did not
waste so much breath, together with pen,
ink and paper, as I had done to expose the
assassin's assertions respecting their *putting
out* Mr. Pitt, which they truly effected.

"That the final order having been given to
put out Mr. Grey by the pneumatic magnetists having in charge the Admiralty Department, for attaining its secrets, actuating
its members, &c. the moment was determined on, and he actuated to be in a given
place by the time. That this being well
known as it proceeded, another magnetist
contrived to puppet one of their prepared
victims to be there also; and the fluid of
this person (a Sir Michael Le Fleming,)
having been rendered more attractive than
Mr. Grey's; the wrench took hold of Sir
Michael instead of Mr. Grey, and killed him

on the spot; while, they say, by the force,
Mr. Grey would have escaped with a rup-
ture like the late Duke of Bedford, or the
bursting of some blood-vessels which would
not have produced death. Then they cried
' *It's yho* (you) *that presearved* (preserved)
him,' in their affected provincial jargon;
for provincial is not their real language.
During some weeks previous to this, they
had been ripping at my ventricles by their
air-loom-force: a dreadful operation it is!
They pretended they worked Mr. Grey into
the foreign office, where he might have the
means of knowing the reality of the ad-
vances made by France to the British Government through *me* in 1793, and the folly
of his chief friend Lord Grenville, thereupon,
and then they said an expert was preparing
a puppet to be actuated commemoratively,
as Lord Grenville and his friends were to be
made to act politically. Every time I saw
the Philanthropic Insurance advertisements

signed William Ludlam, which was daily, *they* would cry ' *Voila le Victime*,' then ' *That's his Ludship, Erskine, Grenville*,' and by brain-saying, refer to Mr. Erskine's mode of speech, for his Lordship pronouncing nearly Ludship, and say that William Ludlam meant William Lud Grenvile, and touching the fluid in my vitals, would make me quite sorry.   When Ludlam, pistol in hand, attempted to tyrant it over the master as well as the waiter of the London Tavern, they said ' *It's exact.   C'est ainsi*,' and to his jumping through the window also, they would cry ' *C'est ainsi aussi*,' and ' *Leighton, Sir William, we puppeted yho, there to commemorate.*'   Some time after, when Ludlam was taken, Lord Erskine ordered him under the care of Dr. Monro, and prohibited the Lord Mayor's warrant from being served against him.   *There* they would cry ' *his Ludship*,' and then brain-say the subject as before.   Then ' *Ween,*

(we will) *puppet yho also,*' and brainsay,
' *We will actuate Erskine Monroish, yet.*'
I mentioned their pretexts and sent out a me-
morandum thereupon, stating that, though
they were active to prevent my perceiving
all their drift, I feared they intended to
make Lord Erskine mad; for they often
asserted, that with but half stress on the
fluid with which he was impregnated, he
would become weak in intellect; and as it
was to my wife, I could not help saying,
' Notwithstanding the readiness to act as
Counsel for me in 1797, which Mr. Erskine
professed, yet, when you called upon him
to ask him from me to mention my case and
imprisonment in Bedlam in the House of
Commons, he would not do so; and for
which the assassins boasted once they stagnated him in the House of Commons, by
an air-loom warp, attaining him from no
great distance; and would have killed him
afterwards there as an example in their pre-

texts but for my exposing their infamous threats; he now cares no more for me than he does for the dogs in the street.' ' *Enough* (they cried) *we'll shew you.*'   At a subsequent time when it was said that the Lord Chancellor, passing along Holborn, saw several persons pursuing and beating a dog in order to kill him, pretending he was mad; '*Aye* , (they cried) *that's as you say we pursue you pelting you with our murdering efforts*;' but he not thinking any madness appeared about him, ran into the midst of them, and taking the dog up in his arms, rescued him from their fury, and ordered him to be conveyed to his stables and taken care of : ' *Yes*, (said they) *that part is the derision of the event ; we have commemorated your words ; he does care about the dog, but you may lie in the stable* (a term used by them for being placed on the incurable establishment in Bedlam) *and be damned.*

" When the change of Ministry came about, then they asked, ' *Now where's poor Ludlom* ?' He was actuated to a thought, that, with pistols pointed to them, he could force the parties to yield to him; but the good sense of the master of the tavern left him no alternative but to jump through the window and be off—brainsaying, that Lord Grenville and Co. were also endeavouring to establish their philanthropic assurance to the Catholics, thinking to make as much more than legal interest thereby, as Lud-lam and his partizans did by their philanthropic assurance, to gain them 8 per cent. besides bonuses frequently; and as Lud-lam had first opponents in his own party or subscribers, and then for his pistolling was forced through the window, so Lord Grenville, after having endeavoured to force the *Master* to comply with his wishes, was in turn forced through the window into the street, a term among them for *turned out.* Lud Erskine and some

others were Lord Grenville and Co's. opponents in the cabinet to the philanthropic
efforts to make more than common interest.
They pretended they worked Ludlam into
Dr. Monro's hands, as completing the event
of my being in them : asserting, that the
working the former Administration out, and
Lord Grenville in, the rendering all their
measures abortive, and then pushing them
on to be turned out, was to commemorate
and retaliate upon them, for their parts in
the persecution and imprisonment I experienced."

SECOND EVENT-WORKING.

" I ought not to omit mentioning, that
about three or four years since, when the
assassins so much boasted that a great deal
of fluid prepared by them was sent to im-
pregnate the *Mollys*, as they termed *Mollen-*

dorf, Brunswick, Kamenskoi, &c. to make
fools of them in the battles the event-
workers were working to produce : they said
Russia must be weighed by me, crying,
' *We told you that you were Buonaparte's
talisman, and that we would work him up
to as high a pitch of grandeur by the possession of you, as we would fix you degraded
below the common level of human nature,*"
(an expression often indeed used by them in
menacing me during the years they so
threatened to murder my son and all my
family, if I would not forgive them : and
would not only counteract me in every thing,
but make every person presenting himself
mock and ridicule me, and kill me at last,
either secretly or openly, for that I should
never escape out of their clutches alive ; and
after having asserted they would bring Russia
to the balances for a few months, they cried
' *Yho are coming,*' brainsaying, that a magnetic fluid impregnated Russian was coming.

Soon it was announced through Bedlam, that some of the Royal Family were coming —preparations were made to receive them, when, lo! as the party entered the gallery, while the assassins were crying, ' *Now for it, we will play you off,*' brain-saying, they should actuate him while they tortured me. One of the patients came to tell me that it was not any of the Royal Family, but the Duke of Somerset and the Russian Ambassador who were coming down. ' *Aye, aye!* (said the assassins) *we told you we would give you notice,*' and began to torture and fluid-lock me, viz. binding all the small nerves and fibres so numerous about the parts composing the root of the tongue, which prevents regularity of speech, and forces me to speak rather slower and to be guarded at every word to prevent stammering. When the party came to my cell, five or six of them, I began to explain to them the manner in which I was assailed, and describe to them the nature of it, enquiring

if they understood Pneumatic Science, &c.
His Grace was with his left arm on the cor-
ner of my bed, and the party generally,
politely attentive; but one of them attracted
my notice from his seeming to become a
little restless, going out of the cell, and not
attending to what I was stating. The assassins said, '*That's the victim.*' A few
days after, I learned that this person was
the Russian Count Pahlin; the assassins
chuckling, often asked me if I remembered
the Russian with arms too short for his person, and an impediment in his speech, saying, '*It will be all over with the Mollys.*'
Every thing was then quiet, but it was not
long before Prussia began to be agitated,
and this brought on the war which beat it
and the Russians out of the field, and left
the Count Pahlin dead upon it."

———————

By this time it is probable that the curiosity of the reader is sufficiently satisfied concerning the mischievous and complicated science of event-working. Although the fable may be amusing, the moral is pernicious. The system of assailment and working events deprives man of that volition which constitutes him a being responsible for his actions, and persons not so responsible, in the humble opinion of the writer ought not to be at large. After the commission of murder or treason, it would be considered an inadequate defence for the perpetrator to alledge that he had been irresistibly actuated by the dexterous manœuvres of Bill, or the Middle man; nor is it at all probable, that the accurate records of Jack the Schoolmaster would be admitted as evidence in a court of law.

There are already too many maniacs allowed to enjoy a dangerous liberty, and the Governors of Bethlem Hospital, confiding in the skill and integrity of their medical officers, were not disposed to liberate a mischievous lunatic to disturb the good order and peace of society. These gentlemen can have no advantage in detaining a person in confinement who has recovered his senses. Their interest consists in the numbers who are restored to the community and their friends; and their only reward the incense which Gratitude projects on the altar of Reason.

FINIS.

LONDON:
Printed by G. Hayden, Brydges Street, Covent Garden.